The Internet for Nurses and Allied Health Professionals

Second Edition

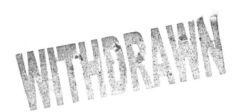
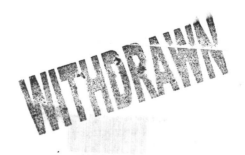

Springer
New York
Berlin
Heidelberg
Barcelona
Hong Kong
London
Milan
Paris
Singapore
Tokyo

Margaret J.A. Edwards, Ph.D., R.N.
Margaret J.A. Edwards & Associates, Inc.
Calgary, Alberta
Canada

The Internet for Nurses and Allied Health Professionals
Second Edition

With a Foreword by Kathryn J. Hannah

With 29 Illustrations

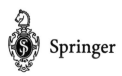 Springer

Margaret J.A. Edwards, Ph.D., R.N.
Margaret J.A. Edwards & Associates, Inc.
52 Canova Road S.W.
Calgary, Alberta T2W 2A6
Canada

Library of Congress Cataloging-in-Publication Data
    Edwards, Margaret J. A.
        The Internet for nurses and allied health professionals / Margaret
    J.A. Edwards. — 2nd ed.
            p.   cm.
        ISBN 0-387-94888-0 (softcover ; alk. paper)
        1. Nursing—Computer network resources. 2. Internet (Computer
    network) 3. Medical care—Computer network resources. 4. Allied
    health personnel. I. Edwards, Margaret J A. Internet for nurses
    and allied health professionals. II. Title.
        [DNLM: 1. Computer Communication Networks—nurses' instruction.
    2. Information Systems—nurses' instruction. 3. Allied Health
    Personnel. W. 26.5 E261 1997]
    RT50.5.E36   1997
    004.67'8—dc21
    DNLM/DLC
    for Library of Congress   96-53902

Printed on acid-free paper.

Production managed by Natalie Johnson; manufacturing supervised by Jeffrey Taub.

Photocomposed copy prepared using the author's Microsoft Word files.

Printed and bound by Edwards Brothers, Inc., Ann Arbor, MI.

Printed in the United States of America.

9 8 7 6 5

ISBN 0-387-94888-0   SPIN 10784185

Springer-Verlag New York Berlin Heidelberg
A member of BertelsmannSpringer Science+Business Media GmbH

Foreword

Isn't technology WONDERFUL? As recently as four years ago, the complexity of communicating with professional colleagues in other time zones and on other continents was so complex and confusing that most health care professionals simply used the international postal system (to call it a postal service would be an oxymoron!). Only a few sophisticated technophiles among the academic elite of health care professions bothered to use the electronic computer networks. Today such communication is commonplace for many health care professionals. This book provides a guidebook for those health care professionals who are new to the information highway.

Perhaps, it is somewhat of an anachronism that this book, presented in a paper based medium, provides a guide to the future electronic medium that may ultimately replace it. Perhaps the authors will next write a multimedia interactive computer program for the material contained in this book.

The authors of this book have provided the novice on the information highway with information about access routes and destinations. The book will also serve as a driving instructor for the novice who wishes to join the queue at the access ramp for the information highway. For the experienced surfer on the Internet this book provides suggestions of byways, short cuts and side routes to explore along the information superhighways.

No one really knows what the future holds. One thing is certain, it will be a very exciting and exhilarating ride for those health care professionals who use this book to accelerate along the information highway.

Welcome to the electronic network of health care professionals!

khannah@acs.ucalgary.ca
KATHRYN J. HANNAH, R.N., Ph.D.
Adjunct Professor,
Department of Community Health Science,
Faculty of Medicine,
The University of Calgary
Calgary, Alberta, Canada

Preface

The INTERNET. Everyone is talking about it. The newspapers report new applications daily. Even the kids at school are connected! But does the Internet offer anything beyond endless shopping at cybermalls, a plethora of computer games or a worldwide club for computer nerds? Is there anything out there for nurses and allied health professionals? YES, there is! That's what this book is all about.

This book is designed as a primer to the Internet for nurses and allied health professionals who have little or no computer experience. In plain language we will describe the Internet and how it works. We'll outline the ways in which the Internet can be a valuable partner in your practice. Information about using various Internet tools will be given. Finally, we've done some of the searching for you and will provide a "catalogue" of Internet resources that we found, with access directions and a brief summary of each resource. We have not attempted to make this catalogue a massive "yellow pages" directory to all health-related sites. Rather, we have identified key sites related to each topic. Sites included are good starting places for searches and generally include links to other Internet resources.

If, in addition to being a health professional, you are a "techie", who is already well-grounded in the fundamentals of the Internet, you will probably find the chapters to be mostly review. However, you'll find the compilation of health-related resources in the catalogue to be valuable. We have also included a reference list of books that we recommend for a more detailed discussion of the Internet.

Health care is changing daily. Nurses and allied health professionals are scrambling to keep up with an ever-changing "healthscape". Traditional methods of formally communicating with peers through conferences, journals and books are not able to provide the answers that health care providers require in a timely manner. When you need to know now how others have dealt with a proposed health care change, you can't wait three months for the next conference or nine months for the book to come out. This is where you discover the real power of the Internet. Your ability to immediately ask questions or exchange ideas with peers around the world gives you the knowledge edge you need to keep your nursing or health care practice professional and progressive.

The INTERNET... How did we ever manage without it!

Contents

Acknowledgments

The preparation and production of any book requires the input of many people. Bill Day and Ken Dreyhaupt at Springer-Verlag graciously provided both support and technical expertise. Special thanks go to Drs. Kathy and Rick Hannah who provided actual content material and also much encouragement. Darren Bierman produced the line art.

I would like to acknowledge the enormous contribution of my husband, Craig Edwards, in supporting the preparation of the manuscript and preparing the camera-ready copy. Special thanks to my mother, Mary Burchell, and sister, Rosemary Burchell, for child-care above and beyond the call of duty! Finally, my thanks to my children for eating a lot of pizza and giving up the computer (and their mother) while the book was prepared. Thank you all!

M.J.A.E.

1
What Is the Internet?

What Is the Internet?

At the most basic level, the Internet is the name for a group of worldwide computer-based information resources connected together. It is often defined as a network of networks of computers. Today, according to the Internet Society, there are more than 30 million sites (computers) connected throughout the world. Every week, it is estimated that over 1 million sites join the Internet.

One of the major challenges in using the Internet is that there is no clear map of how all those networks are connected. There is also no master list of what information or resource is available where! Because there is no overall structured grand plan, the shape and face of the Internet is constantly changing to meet the needs of the people who use it. The Internet can be likened to a cloud in this way; it's amorphous, without boundaries and constantly changing shape and space. Even in the catalogue that we offer in this book, there will be entries whose location has changed from the time we write about them to the time you try to find them according to our instructions.

Although the thought of all those computers joined together is mind boggling, the real power of the Internet is in the people and information that all those computers connect. The Internet is really a people-oriented community that allows millions of people around the world to communicate with one another. Amazingly, people voluntarily share their time, ideas and products, for the most part, without any personal or financial gain. The computers move the information around and execute the programs that allow us to access the information. However, it is the information itself and the people connected to the information that makes the Internet useful and recreational!

Who Owns and Operates the Internet?

The statistics on the massive size and astronomical growth of the Internet would lead us to believe that somewhere there is a superorganization holding it all together. The reality of the Internet organization is very different. The Internet is not "owned" by anyone, in the usual sense of the word. The organizations and individuals that use the Internet manage and pay for their own pieces through a system that looks a lot like anarchy! There are no CEO's or corporate boards of directors, but rather the Internet is "governed" by a loose confederation of users.

Each organization or individual pays for its own computers and networks and co-operates with its neighbour networks to pay for the communication lines that connect them. Regional networks are an example of this type of organization. In my city, several university departments, four major hospitals, and eight community and private sector organizations, each maintaining their own computer systems, have worked together to develop a network connection between them all. This network is called "Agenet". It is used to send information about ageing among the local network members. The expense of developing and maintaining this local network is the responsibility of the members. Grants, tax money, dues, university and corporate monies are funding sources for these local networks. This example is played out millions of times around the world. Leased lines can then connect local networks to each other. Consortiums of local networks and organizations then pool their purchasing power to obtain leased lines and better support for their members. In this way, you can see that it is the often unstated co-operation of organizations and individuals that allows the Internet to function without specific management. The Internet is owned then by nobody and everybody.

In many countries, the "backbone" of the Internet in that country is funded by government organizations. In the United States, the National Science Foundation (NSF) currently funds the backbone. Supercomputer centres were established around the United States by the National Science Foundation in the mid-1980's. To provide universities and research centres around the country with remote access to these supercomputers, the National Science Foundation funded a backbone network (NSFNET) that connected these supercomputer centres. NSF also provided the funding for connections to the backbone for regional networks. In Canada, CA*net Networking Inc. was formed in 1990 to manage the Internet backbone for Canada, appropriately called CA*net. CA*net is run by a group called CANARIE (Canadian Network for the Advancement of Research, Industry and Education).

Although there is no specific governance of the Internet, voluntary coordinating and overseeing of the workings of the networks is done by the Internet Society. The Internet Society fosters the continued evolution of the Internet through education, support for technical development and provision of a forum for exploring new Internet applications. Membership in this non-profit society is open to any organization or individual. Additionally, any network connected to the Internet agrees to the decisions and standards established by the Internet Architecture Board (IAB). Anyone willing to help can participate in the process of setting standards.

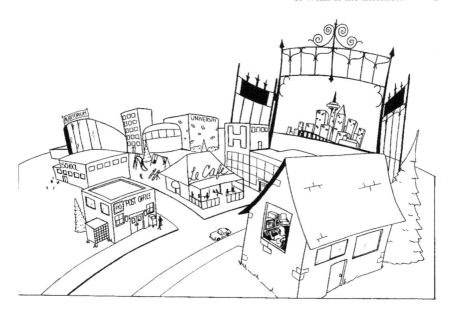

Figure 1.1   An Electronic Town.

What Does the Internet Look Like?

We want to use two analogies that are particularly graphic in describing the Internet: "the electronic town/global village" and "the Information Highway". Figure 1.1 is a graphic representation of an electronic town.

To begin to understand the electronic town, let's start with small town "FreeNets" before we move on to investigate a large metropolis "the Internet". A FreeNet is a computer network that brings together the resources of a community or a campus. Just like most small towns, a FreeNet has a post office where members have mailboxes and can send or receive mail from around the world (electronic mail, called e-mail). There is a town square with small restaurants for one-to-one conversations, and auditoriums or a speaker's corner for large gatherings (places on the network called newsgroups or forums). There's also a gateway that enables users to enter other networks around the world. Other organizations on the network are organizations that exist in the real community; schools and universities, hospitals, newsrooms, weather stations, and libraries. All of this is just a telephone call away using your modem and computer! FreeNets exist in most major cities. The biggest problem with FreeNets is the same problem found in many small towns: there are not enough busses in and out of town! In our city of over 750,000 people, there are only 44 connection lines to the FreeNet. That means a lot of standing in line waiting for the bus! We'll talk about ways other than FreeNets to access the Internet in Chapter 2.

If you've driven around through small towns, you will have noticed that they all have some unique claim to fame; an airplane museum in one, the world's most accurate clock, a database of articles on the mating habits of mosquitoes or the world's biggest supercomputer in others. Imagine the planet covered with those unique little towns and you have a good picture of the Global Village. Rather than having to drive from one town to another, you can travel to any of these towns with your computer via the Information Highway, the Internet, without ever leaving home. You can look at the Monet collection in the Louvre in Paris with as much ease as using the FreeNet to check local library listings.

Where Did the Internet Come From?

The need to transfer information between computers was recognized soon after computers were developed. At first, this type of information transfer was done by putting the information from one computer onto magnetic tape or punch cards (remember, this is in the early 1960s). Then you would carry it to another computer where the information could be loaded from the tape or cards. We still do this today but with files written in ASCII format on a diskette. (This type of a network is called "sneaker net"!). In the 1960's, computer scientists began exploring ways to directly connect remote computers and their users.

In 1969 the U.S. government Department of Defense Advanced Research Projects Agency (ARPA), funded an experimental network called ARPANET. The main goals of the ARPANET research were to link together the Department of Defense and military research contractors that included a large number of universities, and to develop a reliable network. The development of a reliable network involved the concept of dynamic rerouting, which is key to understanding Internet communication today (we'll come back to this concept in Chapter 2). Dynamic rerouting, from the military perspective, would allow communications on a network to be rerouted if part of the network was destroyed by an enemy attack.

The military's goal of a "reliable" network has been accomplished. There are many reports of the Internet being used in "war". Chinese students used their university Internet connections to keep in touch with the world during the Tiannanmen Square uprising. Moscow residents used the Internet to report on events during the attempted overthrow of the government in the Soviet Union. Both civilians and the military used Internet routing technology in the Gulf War and the Bosnian conflict.

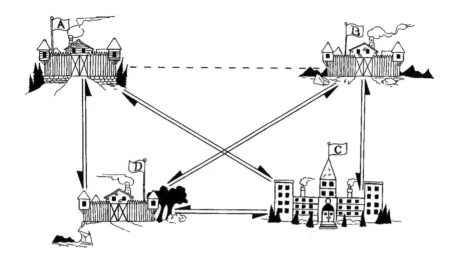

Figure 1.2   Use of Dynamic Rerouting

Figure 1.2 demonstrates the idea of dynamic rerouting. There are normally direct communication links between all four locations, A, B, C and D. In Figure 1.2, the direct link between locations A and B has been severed (more likely by a backhoe than an enemy attack!). A and B cannot communicate directly along the dotted line. However, A can still send messages to B in a number of different ways, as indicated by the solid lines in the figure. For example, the message could be routed from A to D and then to B or from A to C and then to B or from A to D to C and then to B. On the Internet, there is always more than one way for the message to move from you to its intended recipient. This is how ARPANET achieved its goal of developing a reliable network.

The ARPANET became very popular and many universities wanted to join it. To accommodate the growing number of sites, the network also had to be able to add and remove new sites easily and to allow computers of many different types to communicate effortlessly. These needs led to the development of the TCP/IP network protocol. TCP/IP (Transmission Control Protocol/Internet Protocol) is the language that computers connected to the ARPANET used to talk to each other. In the early 1980's all the interconnected research networks were converted to the TCP/IP protocol. The ARPANET became the backbone (physical connection) between all the sites. In the mid 1980's the National Science Foundation established supercomputer centres around the United States. The plan for researchers around the United States to use the ARPANET to connect to those supercomputers did not work out, so the National Science Foundation funded the development of NSFNET. In 1990,

ARPANET was shut down and NSFNET now provides the backbone for Internet communications in the United States.

In Canada, research networking began in the early 1980s. NetNorth, the Canadian equivalent of the American BitNet organization, was created in early 1984. During the period 1985 to 1988, most of the larger universities began multi-year projects to install high speed networks on their campuses. Soon, establishing links between these networks and NSFNET became a priority. At the same time, the National Research Council of Canada developed a plan for the creation of a high speed national network. The University of Toronto, in co-operation with IBM Canada and the telecommunications reseller INSINC, won the contract to build this network. Finally, in June of 1990, CA*net Networking Inc. was formed to manage the Internet backbone in Canada.

What Can I Do with the Internet?

Now that we've briefly described the what the Internet is and where it came from, we want to give you a quick summary of some important Internet resources. All of these resources are discussed in detail in Chapters 3 to 6, but we want you to have a summary of what you can do with the Internet before we get to some of the more technical details in Chapter 2.

Electronic Mail

Electronic mail (e-mail) can be thought of as regular mail-except for the speed of delivery! You can send many of the same things with e-mail as with regular mail—sweaters and jam excepted. Letters, documents, files, data, even sound can be sent via e-mail. While this book was being written, Rick Hannah, who wrote Chapter 8, was in South Africa. Using e-mail, we sent many messages back and forth. Rick e-mailed his chapter and his files with his compiled catalogue listings to be included with the other chapters.

Newsgroups

Newsgroups can be likened to a special interest discussion group. You can participate in discussions about a variety of topics, or you can just "listen in" to the discussion.

Database Searching

In the same way that you conduct a database search in a hospital or university library using CD-ROM technology, you can search data bases through the Internet. You can access many of the same databases, such as Cinahl, as you would through your library, but do it without having to go down to the library and wait your turn.

How Do I Get There from Here?

Now that you have an idea of what the Internet is and what it can do for you, the next chapter describes various ways of connecting to the Internet and getting you on the Information Highway. Who knows, you may find out that you're already connected and didn't know it!

2
How Does the Internet Work?

Connecting to the Internet

If you have access to a telephone line, a modem and a computer, you can connect to the Internet. There are four basic ways to connect to the Internet; make a direct connection over dedicated communications lines; use your computer to connect to a university or hospital computer system that has Internet access; buy time and connections from a commercial Internet service provider; or use an indirect service provider. The next section will describe the various options for connecting to the Internet, including the advantages and disadvantages of each. Then, we'll give some guidelines to help you select the connection that is appropriate for you.

Types of Internet Connections

Direct Connection to the Internet

A direct or dedicated connection wires your computer directly to the Internet through a dedicated machine called a router or gateway. The connection is made over a special kind of telephone line. The gateway makes you an "official" Internet computer that must remain on-line all the time. This type of direct connection is very expensive to install and maintain. For this reason, it is usually used only by large companies or institutions rather than by individuals or small businesses.

Connecting Through Another's Gateway

Another way to connect to the Internet is to use a gateway that another company or institution has established. In this case, a company or university or hospital that has an Internet gateway allows you to connect to the Internet using their system. The connection is usually made through a modem or remote terminal. This type of access is often available to students through the computing services department of their university. Many hospitals and health services organizations also allow staff access to the Internet through the institution's facilities. This is a good way to begin to learn about the Internet resources that are available, before deciding that you want your own access. The only disadvantage is that the institution may not offer full Internet access, but only e-mail and newsgroup facilities. In order to use an institution's access, you will need a login id and password (see Chapter 3). The information services or computer services department is the place to start inquiring about getting access and authorization to the institution's services. For the individual, this is the best type of access to have if full Internet access is available. Someone other than you maintains the computer system, and the Internet connection and, most importantly, pays for the connection. If you have this type of access, celebrate your good fortune!

Connecting Through a Commercial Service Provider

Connecting to the Internet through a service provider is much the same process as using another's gateway. The service provider builds and maintains the gateway and sells Internet connection access to individuals and small companies. Service providers usually charge a flat fee for membership, usually so many dollars per month for so many hours of Internet access per month. Some providers also charge based on the amount of extra time you spend connected to the Net or on the amount and size of e-mail messages that you send. There are also different types of services available through commercial service providers.

Service providers may provide you with a SLIP (Serial Line Internet Protocol) or PPP (Point to Point Protocol) connection. With this type of connection, you dial in to the service provider's computer and connect through the gateway. Your computer, as long as it stays connected, becomes an "official" part of the Internet. With a SLIP or PPP connection, you have full Internet access, up to the power and storage capacity of your own computer. The major disadvantage of using a SLIP or PPP connection is the amount of technical computer expertise that is usually required to install and maintain this type of connection on your computer. Unless you are a computer wizard, this is most likely something that the novice Internet user will want to avoid.

Another service that is available through commercial service providers is called a terminal emulation connection. With this type of service, the provider gives you a simple dial-up program that you can easily install on your computer. When you start up the program, it connects you with the service provider's computer. The service provider's computer then makes the Internet connection. What you see on your screen from then on is only the image of what is really on the service provider's computer. The service provider's computer "paints" your screen to look like its screen. All the "computing" is being done on the service provider's machine and only "reflected" onto your screen. You use your computer to control the actions of the Internet session but your computer is not do-ing any of the intense computing work. This allows you full Internet access even though your own computer would not have the power or storage capacity to provide this on its own. The major advantage to this type of service is that the novice user only needs to load one file from a disk onto their own computer, and the rest of the process is solely "point & click". The internetworking and connection done by the service provider are hidden, making this a very easily accessible type of connection. The disadvantage is that some commercial serv-ice providers who use terminal emulation aren't able to arrange full Internet access, for example, access to the World Wide Web.

Although this section has focused on commercial service providers, many cities and towns also have free community computing services called "FreeNets". These services function much like using another's gateway. The major advantage is they are free. The main disadvantage is that FreeNets do not provide full Internet access. FreeNets generally supply e-mail and newsgroup access but not the ability to search databases or connect to remote host computers.

Connecting Through an Indirect Service Provider

On-line services such as America Online, Compuserve, Delphi and Prodigy have supplied for some time now a place for experimentation with new soft-ware, discussion groups and file transfers. They all now offer Internet access in varying degrees. The advantage again, is that the internetworkings of connecting to the Internet are hidden to the user, so connecting is a simple process. Some of the disadvantages are that full Internet access is not available through all on-line providers, and on-line services fees generally include not only a membership fee but also connect time charges. If you are only going to use the Internet for two to three hours per month this might be an alternative to consider. However, some on-line service providers not only charge for connect time, but also for numbers of characters transferred as files.

What to Look for When Choosing an Internet Provider

These are just a few simple guidelines to keep in mind if you want to pursue getting your own Internet connection. Always remember that it is up to you to be an informed buyer. If a provider doesn't have the time or desire to answer your questions before you buy a service, think about the kind of support you are likely to get from that provider when something goes wrong (end of sermon).

There are several basic elements when you consider getting access to the Internet through a provider. First, what kind of computer do you have to work with? Generally, providers are most comfortable supporting PC-compatible computers. The processing power and storage capacity of your computer are also important. Some of the Internet facilities (i.e., World Wide Web) make strong demands on your computer's resources. Be sure to have this information ready for discussion with a service provider.

Second, what is your own level of technical knowledge and comfort when working with your computer? We're not talking nuclear physics here but it is important to understand that there are many links to this connection chain. You may become involved in levels of technical details that you didn't want to know about. The good news here is that some Internet providers, for a fee, will help you install the connection software on your computer and get it working.

Third, look for a provider with a local telephone number that you use to connect. Some providers advertise 1-800 numbers that you use. The point here is to avoid additional telephone charges. Without a local number, you end up paying additional costs to a telephone company. It can be a dangerous shock to the system to receive a surprise telephone bill after you've been surfing the Net for 20 hours last month.

Fourth, what set of Internet services or tools does the provider offer? You may be perfectly satisfied with just an e-mail account but we seriously doubt it. Be sure to check the details of what is offered and what, if any, additional charges there might be for things such as number of e-mail messages sent, etc.

Fifth, what is the cost of this connection? Be sure that all the restrictions and assumptions are fully identified. One provider we talked to offered unlimited access to the Internet for a really low monthly charge. The hitch was that you were only allowed to be connected for a maximum of 90 minutes in one stretch. After that, you were automatically disconnected. Of course, you could immediately try to dial back in but.... This may be perfectly satisfactory for an infrequent e-mail user but for someone trying to search the Net for information, 90 minutes goes by very quickly (and it usually ends right in the middle of something interesting).

Last, what kind of technical support does the provider offer? If you have trouble coping now when your computer gives you fits, ask some tough questions about the kind and level of support from the provider. Make sure of the support policy of the provider (i.e., 24 hours a day, business hours only, etc.).

The most important thing to keep in mind is that commercial access to the Internet is a fairly new development. There are many new service providers trying to capitalize on the interest about the Internet. A lot of the programs that are used to connect to the Net are still new. A large amount of patience is, we believe, called for. The result of that patience and effort is very rewarding.

Finding Information on the Internet

Internet Addresses

Before you can start to look for information or people on the Internet, it is vital to understand Internet Addressing. Every person and every computer that is on the Internet is given a unique address. Once you know someone's Internet address, you can send mail, transfer files and even have a conversation. When someone wants to tell you where on the Internet certain information about a specific topic can be found, they do it by telling you the Internet address of a computer where the information is stored.

All Internet addresses follow the same format: the person's userid (user-eye-dee) followed by the @ symbol, followed by the unique name of the computer. For example, my university-based Internet address is

marge@cs.athabascau.ca

In this example, the userid portion is **marge** and the unique computer name is **cs.athabascau.ca**. That unique computer name is also called the *domain*. We also have an Internet account with a service provider. That address is

edwardsc@cia.com

and the answer to your question is "No, I don't work for the CIA!" In general, an Internet address has 2 parts, the userid and the domain put together like this:

userid@domain

As you probably can guess, that combination needs to be unique on the entire Internet so that the right person receives your important message!

The domain in an address is actually made up of sub-domains, each one separated by a period. In our first example, the domain is **cs.athabascau.ca** and the sub-domains, from left to right are **cs**, **athabascau** and **ca**. The real way to understand a domain name is to look at the sub-domains in it, reading them from right to left. The rightmost sub-domain is the most general and the sub-domains become more specific as you read to the left. That rightmost sub-domain is called the *top-level domain* and there are 2 different sets of top-level domains. The old-style set is called *organizational domains* and the new style is called *geographical domains*. My two addresses are examples of each style.

Domain	Meaning
at	Austria
au	Australia
ca	Canada
ch	Switzerland ("Confoederatio Helvetia")
de	Germany ("Deutschland")
fr	France
gr	Greece
jp	Japan
us	United States

Table 2.1   Examples of Geographical Top-Level Domains

In the first example, **marge@cs.athabascau.ca**, the most general sub-domain is **ca**. That identifies the computer as being located in Canada (see Table 2.1 for other examples). The next sub-domain identifies the university in Canada where the computer is located, **athabascau**. The last sub-domain, **cs**, identifies the Computer Sciences departmental computer in the university in Canada that holds the mailbox of **marge**.

The second example, **edwardsc@cia.com**, shows the other kind of domain. Instead of first referring to a geographic location (i.e., Canada), the most general part of this domain begins with **com**, identifying this computer system as part of the commercial organization domain. Before the days of international networks, the set of organizational domains (see Table 2.2) was defined mostly for use in the United States. The next sub-domain, **cia**, identifies the name registered on the Internet for a particular company.

Domain	Meaning
com	commercial organization
edu	educational institution
gov	government
int	international organization
mil	military
net	networking organization
org	non-profit organization

Table 2.2   Organizational Top-Level Domains

As a rule, Internet addresses use all lowercase letters. If you see an address with some uppercase letters, it's safe to change them to lowercase. However, if you decide to use uppercase letters, don't use them on the userid as it may make a difference to some computers.

Every person and computer on the Internet has an address. The majority of Internet addresses follow the above format. As a rule, though, rather than worry about addressing format when sending e-mail to someone, simply use the exact address that the person gave you.

3
Using Electronic Mail (E-mail)

Electronic mail (or e-mail) was the first Internet application and is still the most popular one. E-mail is a way of sending messages between people or computers through networks of computer connections. E-mail is not limited to just the Internet. E-mail messages can be moved through gateways to other networks and systems, such as Compuserve or America Online. Many businesses already have an internal e-mail system and, with a little work by the employer, employees can send and receive messages from other businesses via the Internet.

E-mail on the Internet is analogous to the regular postal system but faster in delivery of mail. E-mail combines a word processor function and a post office function in one program. Here's a typical scenario. You start up your e-mail program and use a command to begin a new message. You type the message and identify the recipient's e-mail address and your return address. Then, you "send" your message; this is something like dropping your letter in the regular postbox. The electronic postoffice in your system takes over and passes your message on. Electronic packets of data carry your message towards its ultimate destination mailbox. Your message will often have to pass through a series of intermediate networks to reach the recipient's address. Since networks can and do use different e-mail formats, a gateway at each network will translate the format of your e-mail message into one that the next network understands. Each gateway also reads the destination address of your message and sends the message on in the direction of the destination mailbox. The routing choice takes into consideration the size of your message and also the amount of traffic on various networks. Because of this routing, it will take varying amounts of times to send messages from you to the same person. On one occasion, it might be only a few minutes; on others, it might be a few hours. This can be compared to the situation of taking an airplane to travel from New York to San Francisco at different times. Depending on the amount of passenger traffic at the time that you decide to go, you may be able to take a direct flight with no stops or you may have to be routed from New York to Chicago to Denver to San Francisco. Either way you get to your destination, one route just takes longer than the other.

When your message reaches its destination, the recipient can read the message, respond to you with just a few key strokes, forward your message to someone else, file it, print it or delete it.

Anatomy of an E-mail Message

E-mail messages will always have several features in common regardless of the program used to create the e-mail. A typical e-mail message includes a "From:" line with the sender's electronic address, a date and time line, a "To:" line with the recipient's electronic address, a "Subject:" line, and the body of the message. If there are any spelling or punctuation mistakes in the recipient's address, the message will be sent back to you from the electronic postoffice. The "Subject:" line is the place to give a clear, one-line description of your message. This description is usually displayed when someone checks their e-mail. Then they can decide how quickly they want to read your message!

Many mail programs can automatically attach a signature line at the end of your message. The signature line can include the sender's name, telephone number, postal address and Internet address.

Figure 3.1 contains a sample e-mail message. The format may vary on your system, but the general idea will be the same. In the example, the first line starts with the word "From" This line shows the userid of the person or computer that sent the message. In this case it was **marge@cs.athabascau.ca**.

The "Subject" line tells the recipient what the message is about. Make your subject lines very clear because, when a recipient has dozens of messages, the subject line description is often the basis for deciding what is read first!

```
From:         marge@cs.athabascau.ca (Margaret Edwards)
Subject:      Demonstration message
To:           edwardsc@cia.com
Date sent:    Thu, 6 Apr 95 10:46:48 MDT
Copies to:    marge@cs.athabascau.ca (Margaret Edwards)

This is an example of an e-mail message.
```

Figure 3.1   A Sample E-mail Message

The "To:" line indicates the address to which the message was sent. In the example, the message was sent to our commercial Internet address. If the message had been sent to other people at the same time, their addresses would also appear on this line.

The fourth line is a date/time stamp of when the message was sent. The time will include either a time zone designation (mountain daylight time) or GMT (Greenwich Mean Time) when a standard time reference is needed.

If the message has been copied to others, their addresses will appear after the "Copies to:". Copying or forwarding messages to others is easy to do with most mail programs. For this reason, be very prudent in what you say in a message. You never know where it will end up because you have no control over the message once you have sent it.

Next comes the body of the message. While most e-mail messages are text, if your computer and the recipient's computer have the facilities, you can send data files, sound and visual images via e-mail. In the next section we will outline some of the legal issues surrounding e-mail message contents and discuss some standards of Internet etiquette.

Legal Issues

Privacy, libel and copyright are legal issues that can affect e-mail users. Understand that privacy is not assured with electronic mail. There are no legal requirements that prevent an institution or company from reading incoming and outgoing e-mail messages. If you are using your employer's equipment, this is especially applicable. In addition, once you have sent a message, you have no control over what the recipient may do. He may send a copy to someone else without your knowledge. Also, don't assume that messages you receive are private. The sender may have sent that same message to others without using the "Copies to:" function. A final note about privacy: even though you have deleted a mail message from your mailbox, don't assume that it has been completely erased. Many institutional and company policies require regular back-ups of their computer system disks, which generally hold incoming and outgoing mail messages. It is possible that a copy of your message was taken during a regular system backup. Be aware that your e-mail records can be subpoenaed.

A second legal issue for e-mail users is libel. Libel is applicable within e-mail messages and newsgroups (see Chapter 4). Take care with your comments. What you say can be held against you.

Finally, copyright law applies to transferring files and information. It is illegal to distribute copyrighted information by any means, including elec-tronic transfer. It is not uncommon to find material that has been scanned by a user for personal use and then distributed through e-mail. Unless the copyright owner has granted specific permission for the transfer of such material, it is illegal to do so.

E-mail Etiquette

Many of the people that you communicate with over the Internet will never meet you. Their impressions about you will come entirely from the tone, style and content of your messages. There are several Rules of the Road for using the Information Highway.

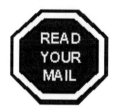

Many people don't have a regular routine of reading their e-mail. This allows messages to build up, often at a great rate! When you finally do sit down to read your e-mail, you may have hundreds of messages. Not only is this taxing on you, it is rude to the senders of those messages. You may miss something important by not keeping up with your mail. If you are getting mail that you don't want, inform the senders that you want your name taken off their distribution list.

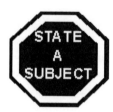

When sending messages, always include a clear description of the message on the subject line. This practice is great for helping you to crystallize your thoughts and express your key idea clearly at the beginning of your message. This courtesy allows recipients to prioritize the order in which they read and respond to their e-mail. It also keeps you from long, run-on messages that have people asking, "What was the question again?"

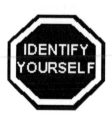

Don't assume that the recipient of your message can figure out who you are from the information in the "From:" line. Be sure to give any contact information that you want the recipient to have. Some people copy a short standard personal identification file into their messages to make this easier, i.e., a signature line.

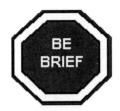

E-mail messages often tend to be "stream of consciousness" based. They ramble on as you try to put your thoughts together while you are responding. Take time to organize your messages or responses before you begin to enter them. Your recipients will appreciate the succinctness of your messages. This will help build you a positive Internet reputation.

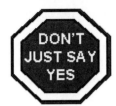

Nothing is more frustrating than receiving an e-mail message that says "yes." You're left wondering which of the six questions you originally posed is being answered. You know how that makes you feel, so don't do it to others. Always include the question to which you're replying in a brief form.

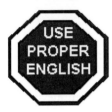

A message full of spelling and punctuation errors reflects badly on you. Ensure that your e-mail messages are properly spelled, punctuated and grammatically correct. This may be the only time that people "see" you. Be sure to make a good impression. For convenience, there are a number of widely used abbreviations found in Internet communications, including

Abbreviation	Meaning
BTW	By The Way
IMHO	In My Humble Opinion
TIA	Thanks in advance
FWIW	For What It's Worth

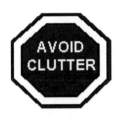

When replying to a message, unless it is REALLY necessary, avoid including the previous message. The Information Highway is often backlogged with volumes of unnecessary information. Don't contribute to this cluttering problem. In the same way, avoid copying the message to a long list of users who are either marginally interested or completely uninterested in what you are sending. Also avoid including a request for automatic confirmation of receipt of the message unless it is vital to have one. Since many mailing packages require only a quick click of the mouse to request confirmation of receipt and then confirmation of reading, users get carried away checking off these and many other unnecessary options. The result is several "confirming" messages being sent for every one real message. Unless the message is urgent, avoid tagging it as such.

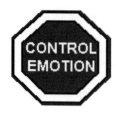

Although e-mail allows easy expression of ideas, it does not allow the recipient of your message to hear the tone of your voice or see the body language that accompanies your message. Be careful, for example, in how you express anger through your message. Because e-mail is faceless, many people seem to lose their inhibitions and feel that they can say exactly what they want (but probably shouldn't!). Angry blasts meant for one person are often forwarded to others and used against you. Often in written messages it's difficult to identify humor or sarcasm. Use a "smiley" to convey your emotions. Smileys are an example of "emoticons", icons for indicating emotions. Turn your head sideways to see them: :-) (Happy Smiley), :-((Sad Smiley) or 8-) (Smiley with glasses). There's got to be a bit of fun in all this serious message-sending! And finally, DON'T SHOUT. Typing your message in all capital letters is like shouting. Use capital letters SPARINGLY, only for emphasis.

Mailing Lists

Mailing lists are an extension of e-mail. When you send an e-mail message to someone, you indicate his or her address. When you consistently want to mail to the same group of people, you can set up a special recipient name called an *alias*. For example, a hospital could create an alias called "nursing" that lists the e-mail addresses of all the directors of nursing. To send a message to all the directors of nursing, you simply specify "nursing" in the "To:" line and the same message will be sent to everyone on that list (alias). The directors of nursing can use this method to have an electronic discussion group. One director sends a message about a certain topic that is distributed to all those users identified by the alias "nursing" (all the other directors of nursing). When another director wants to respond to the topic, a message is sent again to "nursing" and all the directors of nursing receive it.

A mailing list is like an alias that contains hundreds or thousands of users from all over the Internet. Any message sent to the mailing list "alias" will automatically be sent to everyone on the mailing list. Everything that anyone says through the mailing list goes to everyone on the mailing list. Mailing lists facilitate electronic discussion groups. Each mailing list resides at a specific computer and is looked after by a human administrator. The host computer is responsible for distributing incoming messages to all mailing list members. The administrator is responsible for maintaining the mailing list. Some mailing lists are also moderated. In these lists, there is a moderator who reviews each incoming message for appropriateness and either passes it through for distribution or rejects it. Some moderators will also prepare *digests*, something like an issue of a magazine. The digest will be a whole set of messages and articles in one package, making it much easier to keep up with the messages.

These mailing lists are maintained in two ways, either manually by a person or by a program. In the manual approach, the list administrator takes care of adding or deleting addresses from the master distribution list. In the program approach, you send messages to the address of a computer that provides this service. The most common mailing list administration program is called *Listserv* (standing for **List server**). Many of the mailing lists in our catalogue are maintained by "Listserv" systems. We'll describe the ways of subscribing and unsubscribing to mailing lists in the next section.

Subscribing, Unsubscribing and Mailing to Mailing Lists

Mailing lists are traditionally organized around specific topics. Many of these are profession or occupation-specific. For example, NURSENET is a mailing list that hosts general discussion about nursing. Other examples of profession-specific mailing lists include GradNrse, MEDLAB-L (for Medical Laboratory Technology), and Psychiatric Nursing List. These and others of interest to health care professionals are found in the catalogue section of this book.

As we described in the previous section, mailing lists are administered by either by a person or by a program. In either case, you subscribe or unsubscribe to a list by sending an e-mail message to a specific address. This address will be for the administrator of the list, whether human or machine. The format for most subscribe/unsubscribe messages to a list administrator follows a similar format.

As an example of an automated mailing list, to subscribe to NURSENET, you send an e-mail message to LISTSERV@LISTSERV.UTORONTO.CA. By the address, you can see that this is an automated list (the address LISTSERV gives it away). For subscribe and unsubscribe messages, the "Subject:" line is ignored so you don't put anything in it. However, in the body of the message, you must put, on a line by itself, the command

SUB NURSENET <first name> <last name>

where the <first name> and <last name> are your first and last names. After a period of time, you'll receive a confirmation message that you are subscribed. Shortly after that, you'll begin receiving messages from the list. You can unsubscribe in the same way with the UNSUB command but you don't have to enter your name. The line in the body would look like

UNSUB NURSENET

Listserv machines have other commands to give you control of the messages you receive. To get a list of available commands, send a message to the listserv machine with the word HELP, on a line by itself, in the body of the message. A return message will give you a complete command set.

A list maintained by a person is fairly easy to spot by its address since the address will contain "-REQUEST". For example, the list, PHARM (for Pharmacology), gives instructions to send a SUBSCRIBE message (same format as for the above Listserv example) to:

PHARM-REQUEST@DMU.ac.uk

This tells you that a human will respond to your request for subscription.

Once you have subscribed to any of these lists, you will receive instruction on what address to send messages to if you want those messages "posted to the list" (i.e., have a copy of your message sent to all addresses on the mailing list).

Mailing List Etiquette

There are a few additional points of etiquette that apply to mailing lists specifically. Most of them have to do with reducing the amount of unnecessary messages on the Net. It is important to remember that the resources of the Internet are not infinite. If people on the Net do not take responsibility for "conserving the environment", so to speak, all users will suffer.

The first point is common sense. When you first get on the Net, it is very tempting to join many different mailing lists because they all sound so interesting. That's true. They are interesting, and hundreds of people read them and respond daily. But the number of messages generated from even one mailing list can be overwhelming. Try joining mailing lists one at a time. Monitor how much information comes from a list and whether you really want to be on this list. As we said earlier, you need to have the time to read your mail so choose your lists carefully.

Once you've joined a mailing list, spend some time *lurking*. Lurking means just listening in on the group discussion without replying. This will allow you to discover the tone of the group, the types of topics covered, and current topics of conversation. Asking questions or making comments immediately upon joining a group, without knowing the culture, can result in angry censoring by the group. One of the most important sources for topics and purpose of the list can be found in the FAQ (Frequently Asked Questions). It is a list of questions and answers that is regularly posted on a list to help newcomers understand what this particular list is all about. Find it on your list and read it.

A sure sign of a newcomer is a message sent to the list "just to see if it works." Even though the subject line may say "Test message, please ignore", it can still annoy a lot of people. Don't forget that a message posted to the list means that message is sent to **all** the addresses on the list.

Along that same thought, be careful in how you respond to a question that someone posts to the list. You may have an answer but it is better to send that answer in a message to the **person** who asked the question rather than post the answer to the list. If several people respond to the originator, it is more efficient and effective for the originator to summarize the answers and post them once to the list.

Finally, we want to reinforce the importance of how you present yourself through your messages. When you send a message to a friend, they will make allowances for you because they know you. When hundreds of people all over the world are reading your responses, take the time to use correct spelling, punctuation and grammar. Present yourself well, someday you may meet some of these people face to face.

4
Newsgroups

Discussions take place on the Internet using both mailing lists and newsgroups but there is a significant difference between the two methods. A mailing list discussion comes directly to your electronic mailbox, just like a letter is delivered by a postal service. However, the messages that form discussions in newsgroups are only sent to the newsgroup administrator, who then sends them to Internet newsgroup system sites (not individual subscribers). You then read the messages in the newsgroup at a particular system site just as you would walk down the hall to read the messages posted on a bulletin board. In fact, the origin of newsgroups was as a bulletin board service where messages could be posted for all to see. In summary, instead of the messages coming directly to you via a mailing list, you go to a place where the messages are posted in a newsgroup and read them there.

What Is Usenet?

Usenet (User's Network) is made up of all the machines that receive network newsgroups. A machine that receives these newsgroups is called a Usenet Server. Any computer system that wants to carry newsgroups of interest to that site can be a Usenet server. If you are affiliated with an institution, it is probably a Usenet site. Ask your system administrator! If you have your own Internet access through a service provider, ask that provider about the newsgroups that it carries.

Instead of forwarding all messages to all users on a mailing list, Usenet forwards all messages (called *articles* to keep up the newspaper analogy) not to individual subscribers, but to other Usenet servers who forward them on until all machines that are part of Usenet have a copy of your article (message). Individuals then use programs called "newsreaders" to access the newsgroup through their own computer.

A typical Usenet server receives more than 20,000 articles per day. To organize all these articles, they are assigned to specific newsgroups. Newsgroups are further collected into hierarchies, similar to the domains described in relation to e-mail addresses. Table 4.1 shows an example of some of the most important Usenet newsgroup hierarchies.

Name	Topic
alt	alternative newsgroups
bionet	biology
biz	business, marketing, advertisements
comp	computers
k12	kindergarten to grade 12
misc	anything that doesn't fit into another category
news	about Usenet itself
rec	recreation, hobbies, the arts
sci	science of all types

Table 4.1 Example of Usenet Newsgroup Hierarchies

Every Usenet server subscribes to specific newsgroups. Not all newsgroups are available on all Usenet servers. Again, you will have to ask your system administrator or service provider for a list of newsgroups to which your system subscribes.

Some newsgroups are moderated. This means that you cannot post articles directly to the newsgroup. Instead, all messages sent to this newsgroup will be automatically routed to the volunteer moderator. The moderator then decides what articles to send on to the newsgroup. Articles may be edited by the moderator or grouped with other articles before they are forwarded to the newsgroup. In some cases, the moderator may decide not to forward an article at all. Moderators exist to limit the number of low-quality articles in a newsgroup, especially all those "me too" or "I agree" type of articles.

Components of a Usenet Article

Messages sent to a newsgroup are called articles. Just like an e-mail message all articles have common features. Each article begins with a header. The header, which may be up to twenty lines long, contains technical information about the article. The body of the article follows. The same Rules of the Road that we discussed in Chapter 3 apply when sending articles to Usenet newsgroups. Finally, a signature block is placed at the end of your article. Although your name will appear in the header, a signature block with at least your name and e-mail address is standard. Many users place quotations or small graphics on their signature line.

In Figure 4.1, you can see that there are individual articles (e.g. "Acid Reflux") and that the moderator has grouped some articles together (e.g. "Bad Breath"). The numbers in the square brackets tell you how long the individual article is (i.e., "Acid Reflux" is 10 lines long) or how many articles are in each group (i.e., "Bad Breath" has 5 articles). The name of this newsgroup is **misc.kids.health**.

misc.kids.health			
📄 "The perfect food"	[44]	04/05	Bryan J. M
📄 Acid Reflux	[10]	04/04	Ken Solon
📄 Atrial Septal Defect -- Anybody been throu	[20]	04/04	Lenore Ma
📁 Bad Breath	[5]		
📁 Chicken Pox Twice in a Month	[4]		
📁 goomy eyes	[2]		
📁 Growing up connected to nature	[3]		
📄 gummy eyes	[8]	04/05	Laura Joh
📄 Labial adhesions	[18]	04/05	Nancy@du

Figure 4.1   Example of Articles Found in a Newsgroup

Joining a Newsgroup

When you first join or subscribe to a newsgroup, it is advisable to initially spend time *lurking* (discussed in Chapter 3). You will want to monitor the articles in the group for a while to see what the tone of the group is (are the articles academic in tone or informal?), who the regular participants are, and what types of topics are discussed. Most news groups have an FAQ (Frequently Asked Questions) file that is well worth reading before you start asking questions that will reflect badly on you!

Another resource to explore is a special newsgroup for new users of Usenet called **news.announce.newusers**. Articles that appear on this newsgroup include:

- rules for posting to Usenet
- how to work with the Usenet community
- FAQ's about Usenet
- Emily Postnews on Netiquette
- Writing style for Usenet

Reading Articles

In order to read the articles posted to a newsgroup, you use a program called a newsreader. A newsreader is the interface to Usenet that allows you to choose the newsgroups to which you wish to belong, or select and display articles. Using a newsreader, you can also save articles to a file, mail a copy to someone else or print them. Responding to the article's author or the newsgroup is also done through the newsreader program.

There are a number of common newsreader programs: **rn**, **trn**, **nn**, and **tin**. If your system is a Usenet site, it will also have a newsreader program in place. Talk with your system administrator about the specific newsreader program. The commands used by the various programs are not consistent, so it doesn't make sense to present a large amount of information on each newsreader in this book. Your system administrator can give you the documentation to use the particular newsreader on your system. If you are purchasing your Internet connection from a service provider, they also will have selected a newsreader for use on their system. The service provider can give you the necessary documentation to make the program work for you.

Posting Articles

After you've been lurking for a while, you will decide that you have something to say to the newsgroup to which you've subscribed. Before you reply to an article, determine if your response would be best sent to the author of the previous article or to the entire newsgroup.

Once you've decided where to direct your message, your specific newsreader program will have a number of functions to assist you in sending your own article. Again, as those functions vary with the newsreader program, we will not list them all here, but will direct you to the documentation provided for your system's newsreader.

Don't try a test message to the newsgroup. The people who spent valuable time and money to download your file that says "this is a test" will be less than amused with you and may send unpleasant remarks your way! There are several newsgroups designed to test whether or not your messages are getting through: **misc.test** and **alt.test**. When these newsgroups receive a posting from you, they will automatically send a reply to tell you that you were successful in sending your article. Use these newsgroups to perfect your article-sending skills first.

Final Thoughts

Newsgroups and mailing lists exemplify the power of the Net. You have the ability to call on the resources and creativity of people around the world to help you. As well, you can contribute your experience and share your knowledge with others. This borderless Global Village is the true spirit of the Internet.

5
Telnet and FTP: Remote Login and Retrieval of Information

The Internet can make it as easy to use a computer on the other side of the world as it is to use your own computer. You use a special program called *telnet* to connect to a remote computer (called a *host*). You can then use that computer as easily as if you were using a terminal in the room next to it. You may need an account or a password to connect to that computer. Telnet acts as a go-between for your computer and the other computer. Whatever you type on your computer keyboard is passed on by telnet to the other computer. Whatever is displayed on the other computer screen is passed back to your computer and appears on your computer screen. Your screen and keyboard appear to be connected directly to the other computer. Telnet is also used as a verb. When the local computer network access to my university is not working, I can often "telnet" directly to the university computer system using my commercial Internet account.

Now that you know what telnet is, you will probably want to know what you can do with it. Why would you want to log into other computers, and what would you get once you were logged in? Good questions. When you connect to a remote host through telnet, what you get depends solely on what the host computer provides. Some host resources are similar to bulletin boards, others provide information of specific areas, and still others provide services such as weather reports or games.

To access a remote computer, you will need its telnet address, sometimes the same as its e-mail address but not always. Generally, if a remote computer allows telnet connection, the address is not freely distributed for security reasons. When you start up the telnet program, enter the address of the host computer and the program will attempt to connect you. If your connection fails it may be that: you spelled the address wrong; the host computer is temporarily unavailable (usually for repair work or upgrading); or because of security restrictions. Once you are connected, you enter your userid and password that was given to you for this computer. Some remote hosts offer a public service. If you are accessing one of these types of hosts, often the program starts by itself, without the need to enter a userid or password.

Once your userid and password have been validated, you can take advantage of all the resources provided by the host computer. When you are finished with the remote host, you just issue the *logout* command. This will break the connection and telnet will stop automatically.

For example, you can telnet to a host called **ajn.org** (American Journal of Nursing). You can log in as a NEW user and the system will ask for identifying information, i.e., first name, last name, address, and a password of your choice. Once you are logged in, a menu allows you the choices you see in Table 5.1.

AJN Network	Communication Centre
Internet Newsgroups	Utilities
Nursing Associations	The Lounge
	News Stand

Table 5.1 Menu Choices at **ajn.org**

If you select "News Stand", you get another set of choices as seen in Table 5.2. If you select any of these choices, you get an on-line display of a document.

AJN Newsline	Interactive Newsletter	Healthcare
Press Releases	New Scan	
Hospice Newsletters		

Table 5.2 Menu Choices from "News Stand" Option

FTP

FTP (File Transfer Protocol) is technically the set of specifications that support Internet file transfer. Practically, however, FTP is used to refer to a service that allows you to copy a file from any Internet host to another Internet host (usually your computer). Therefore, FTP is another Internet application that allows you to access a remote host computer. Telnet allows you to log in directly to the remote computer, making your own computer a terminal of the host. FTP, however, only allows you to look at the file names on a remote computer and then copy (download) them to your computer. On some remote sites, you can also upload to the host computer, but you can't "work" on the remote host. FTP is one of the most widely used Internet services. All types of information and computer software are available on the Internet, and FTP lets you copy these onto your own computer. The possibilities are endless: statistics programs, computer games, text files, sound and even video clips.

The only problem is that you must have a valid userid and password to access the remote host and copy files, just as you needed for telnet. If you have an account on the remote host, you can use FTP to log in to your account and then download or upload files between the remote host and your own machine. To facilitate the distribution of information on the Internet, many computers have been set up to be an *Anonymous FTP host*. The systems administrator of an Anonymous FTP host designates specific directories as open to the public and creates a user login called *anonymous* (or sometimes *guest*). Anyone who wants to can log in to that computer with the userid *anonymous* and their e-mail address as the password. You can then copy out any of the files found in the public directories. Those directories, though, are the only ones that the user *anonymous* can see. All other files and directories on the computer are invisible and not accessible. For example, personnel files, research data files and licensed software are kept out of the public directories.

Most computers on the Internet that you can access with telnet or FTP use the UNIX operating system. UNIX is known for its rather cryptic commands. Happily, with the development of graphical user interfaces, many telnet and FTP programs are available that reduce or eliminate the need to learn UNIX commands to run the process. Many of the available windows-based Internet programs allow you to use FTP with a simple "point and click" and make the whole process so easy that you will wonder what all the fuss was about.

Locating Files Using Archie

One of the biggest problems on the Net though is knowing where to find that certain file that you want to copy. After all, there are more than 4 million computers on the Net today. Although there is no single registry of all resources on the Internet, information retrieval systems provide a good way to locate specific information. *Archie* was the first of the information retrieval systems to be developed. The purpose of Archie is to create a central index of files that are available on *Anonymous FTP sites* around the Internet. This is a constantly growing index. To share the demands of many people searching for files, several Archie servers have been created. These are computers whose main job is to periodically connect to participating anonymous FTP sites and download lists of all the files that are on each site. The lists of files are then compiled into a database that you can then search in many ways. In order to use Archie, you must either have an Archie server on your system or use telnet to connect to an Archie server. If you are using the computer facilities of a university, hospital or company, ask your system administrator if you have an Archie server.

One of the drawbacks to this retrieval system is that Archie only collects file names. In order to search the database, you must know at least part of the file name that you are looking for. For example, suppose we were looking for a copy of the program, EpiInfo, a statistical analysis software package.

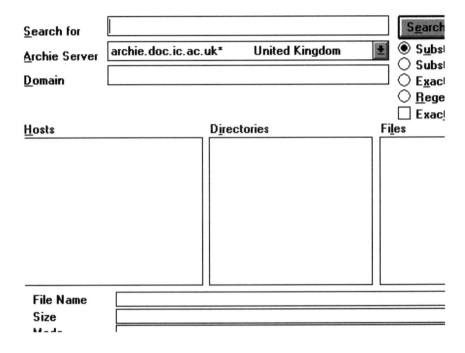

Figure 5.1 Example of an Archie Search Facility

Figure 5.1 is an example of an Archie search facility. Note that the search took place on the Archie server called **archie.doc.ic.ac.uk**. This server was chosen from a list of Archie servers that appears when Archie is invoked. We typed in "epiinfo" on the "Search for" line and pressed the "Search" button. The Archie server came back with a list of the locations of all the files that it knows about called "epiinfo" as shown in Figure 5.2

Once the Archie server has provided you with the location of files that match your search string, you can choose what you want. Then you can use the FTP program to connect to the appropriate machine and download those files that you have selected.

Search for	epiinfo		Sear
Archie Server	archie.doc.ic.ac.uk*	United Kingdom	⊙ Sul
			◯ Sul
Domain			◯ Exa
			◯ Re:
			☐ Exa

Hosts	Directories	Files
ftp.umu.se	/pub/pc/epi	epiinfo
	/pub/pc/epi/epiinfo	

File Name	DIRECTORY: epiinfo
Size	512 bytes
Mode	drwwwwww ..

Figure 5.2 Result of Archie Search for "epiinfo"

In summary, Archie provides an excellent way of locating copies of a particular file that you want. It provides the computer name and directory location of the file. You can then use FTP to retrieve a copy of the file. The unfortunate part of Archie is that it only knows about file names.

The next chapter will examine other information retrieval systems that try to provide some idea of the contents of the files.

6
Finding Information on the Internet

There are many ways to think about information and so there are many ways to categorize and retrieve it. In this chapter, we will introduce you to a number of information retrieval systems: Gopher, Veronica, Jughead, WAIS, and Web browsers. You will want a basic understanding of the entire list of information retrieval tools so that when you have a specific need, you are able to use the right tool for the job. Imagine trying to put a screw into the wall using the blunt end of a knife. It may work, but it definitely takes longer and provides more frustration than if you used a screwdriver. Choose the right tool for the job!

The Gopher

Any of these information retrieval tools can best be understood as part of an on-going evolutionary process. FTP allowed you to browse through the files of a remote host site. This took a great deal of time and the results were haphazard and much less than thorough. For success, you had to already know the file name you needed and which computer to try looking on. Archie was an answer to this problem. With an Archie server, you could specify a file name to use to search all FTP sites. The problem then with Archie was that you didn't always know what the contents of the file were simply by looking at the name of a file. *Gopher* was the answer to that problem.

Gopher was developed to help you to know what is in each file. This is accomplished by an administrator at each site that is a designated *Gopher site*. The administrator starts by examining the contents of all files at that Gopher site. Each file is then categorized in one or more ways. By looking at all the categories, the administrator can group files together. Those groupings form Gopher menu pages. Each file in the group is an item on the menu page and has a descriptive title line. Often the menu pages can be arranged in a hierarchical fashion. The administrator then builds links between the menu pages to reflect this hierarchy.

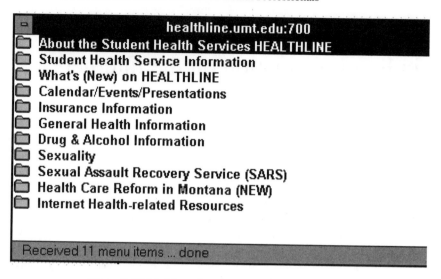

Figure 6.1 Main Menu Page of HEALTHLINE Gopher

Figure 6.1 is the main Gopher menu page at the Healthline Gopher site. Each item on this page represents a link to a sub-menu page. For example, when you select the item "General Health Information", you get the menu as illustrated in Figure 6.2.

The first four items are again links to more sub-menu pages. The other items such as "Asthma" are documents that you can read.

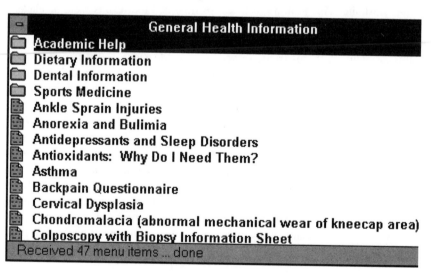

Figure 6.2 Example of Sub-menu Gopher Page

This is only the first screen of the sub-menu under "General Health Information". There is a total of 47 items on this sub-menu. You can see the rest by moving down the page.

All Gopher servers are registered with a main Gopher site at the University of Minnesota, the originator of Gopher. Although much folklore exists about the name, the gopher is the mascot of the University of Minnesota, and was chosen as the name by the program originators.

Gopher Searching

You can find information at a Gopher site by personally browsing through many layers of menus until you find what you want. An analogy would be if you were looking for information about *anonymous* in this book, with only the chapter titles and no index available. You would have to make predictions about which chapter you thought that information would be in. Then you would have to skim through the entire chapter to see if the information really was in that chapter. If it wasn't, then you would make another "guess" and try again. That's how Gopher works. You "flip" through menu pages selecting items that you think might lead you to where you want to go. If you don't want to go anywhere, Gopher is a terrific way to page through and serendipitously find all kinds of interesting (and sometimes even useful) information on the Internet.

Eventually, people became tired of paging through menus and decided that a better search tool was needed. Using the book analogy, it would be the same as reading through a few chapters and not finding what you want. So you give the book to an assistant with instructions to find the information. That assistant is analogous to the information retrieval system called *Veronica* (yes..to keep Archie company).

Veronica and Jughead Searching

Veronica is a program that searches all gopher sites on a regular basis and takes copies of all the items on all their menu pages. Veronica then indexes the key word in each menu item. When you do a Veronica search, you search by key word through all of *gopherspace* (the sum of all Gopher menu items of all Gopher sites in the world). This tool makes finding information at Gopher sites a very simple process. However, if you want to find information from a specific Gopher site, Veronica may not be the right tool for the job.

Jughead was created to search by key word in the menus and sub-menus of a specific Gopher site only. Jughead allows you to select the Gopher site and then specify the search terms. Jughead will then search and retrieve information that is located on the Gopher server that you selected.

WAIS

Another information retrieval program is *Wais* (Wide Area Information Servers, pronounced wayz). Wais can search any of hundreds of collections of data (called a source) that have been stored as Wais documents. You specify the name of the source and the keywords that you want to search. Wais then searches the sources that you specified. One of the advantages of Wais is that it searches the actual contents of documents, not just the document name. Problems arise with Wais if you don't know what source to specify or if Wais doesn't access the source that you want. Also, because Wais searches for any occurrence of the key word you specify, if the key word has more than one contextual meaning, you may get many search items that have no relevance to your real request. If you do not have windows application software on your computer, Wais is very difficult to use. With windows-based software, it is much less difficult. Wais is not one of the most popular information retrieval systems, largely because of the limited number of sources and the past difficulty with non-windows based access. If the source that you wish to search is available to Wais and you have a windows-based application, Wais can provide an excellent way to accomplish an in-depth search of Wais documents.

World Wide Web

The latest service to be developed in the evolution of attempts to make sense of all the Internet resources is the *World Wide Web* (variously called WWW, W3 or the Web). The goal of WWW development was to offer a simple, consistent and intuitive interface to the vast resources of the Internet. WWW tries to provide you with the intuitive links that humans make between information, rather than forcing you to think like a computer and speculate at possible file names and hidden sub-menus as do the previous services. A short history of the development of the WWW will help you understand its services.

History of the Web

In 1989, researchers at CERN (the European Laboratory for Particle Physics) wanted to develop a simpler way of sharing information with a widely dispersed research group. The problems they faced are the same as those you face in using the previous information retrieval systems. Because the researchers were at distant sites, any activity such as reading a shared document or viewing an image required finding the location of the desired information, making a remote connection to the machine containing the information and then downloading the information to a local machine. Each of these activities required running a variety of applications such as FTP, Telnet, Archie, or an image viewer. The researchers decided to develop a system that would allow them to access all types of information from a common interface without the need for all the steps required previously. Between 1990 and 1993, the CERN researchers developed this type of interface, WWW, and the necessary tools to use it. Since 1993, WWW has become one of the most popular ways to access Internet resources.

Hypertext

To navigate around the World Wide Web, you must have a beginning understanding of *hypertext*. Hypertext is text that contains links to other data. For example, when you are doing a literature search using the hard copy of CINAHL, you choose your first search term and look it up. As you read through the listings, another idea for a search term comes to you. You put your finger in the first page (so you can return there easily) and turn to the new term. At the bottom of the listings of the second term is a note that says "see also" and gives you several other words to follow. In a hypertext document, you don't have to wait until the end to find the links, they may be anywhere in the document. Links in hypertext documents are marked either with color bars, underlining or use of square brackets with numbers, so that they stand out. Whenever you read a word that is marked as hypertext, you can select it and immediately the link will take you to another document related to the word or phrase. When you have finished looking at the linked document you simply go back to the previous text, where the program has kept its finger in the page.

This is what makes the Web so powerful. A link may go to any type of Internet resource. For example, the link can take you to a text file, a Gopher site, a Telnet session, or a UseNet newsgroup. Another powerful feature of the Web is that hypertext allows the same piece of information to be linked to hundreds of other documents at the same time. The links can also span traditional boundaries. A hypertext document related to a specific professional group may contain links to information in many different disciplines.

For example, in Figure 6.3, the text "Student Health Services" is underlined. If you selected that text, you would next see the Web page that describes Student Health Information. Chances are that Web page would in reality be the Gopher menu that you found earlier (see Figure 6.1). If you selected "Headaches", you would be linked to an on-line document about headaches and headache management.

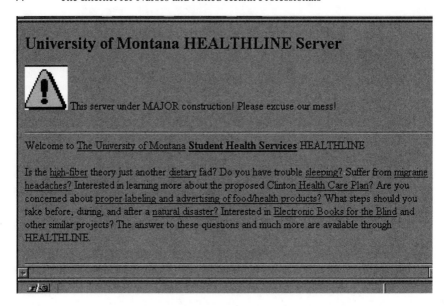

Figure 6.3 The Web Home Page of Healthline

Web Browsers

To access the Web, you will need a Web browser program on your (or your institution's) computer. A Web browser program knows how to interpret and display the hypertext documents that it finds on the Web. There are many browsers on the market. Graphical user interface (GUI) or windows-based browsers include *Netscape*, *Mosaic* and *Cello*. To use these browsers, the hypertext links are highlighted and you simply "point and click" with your mouse. There are also text-based browsers such as *Lynx*. With a text-based browser, each link is given a number enclosed in a square bracket [3]. To select a link, you simply enter the number of the link you want. Regardless of the type of browser you have, navigating the Web is easy and intuitive.

All Web sites have a welcome page, called a home page, that you see when you first connect to that site. The home page may just give the name of the site but usually contains a list of resources and links available at the site.

The World Wide Web project also developed a standard way of referencing an item whether it was a graphics file, a document or a link to another site. This standardized reference is called a *Uniform Resource Locator* (URL). The URL is a complete description of the item including its location. A typical URL is:

http://healthline.umt.edu:700

The first part of the URL, that ends with the colon, is the protocol that is being used to retrieve the item. In this example, the protocol is HTTP (hypertext transfer protocol), used for the Web. Other protocols are self-evident: gopher for Gopher sites, FTP for FTP sites and so on. The next part is the domain name of the computer that you need to connect to (**healthline.umt.edu**). This tells you that the information is on a computer in the education top-level domain (**edu**). The computer is located at the University of Montana (**umt**) and the server name is **healthline**. Most Web browsers will automatically add the "http://" if you simply type the other part of the URL.

Each of the over 30 million Web pages and the additional 1 million added each month, have a unique URL. Finding what you want can be daunting. Search sites are the answer to finding the information "needle" in the WWW "haystack"!

Search Sites

Search sites bring millions of hypertext pages, with their images and multimedia elements into an orderly and searchable structure. Software agents or "spiders" are sent out by search sites to electronically "crawl" the Web, collecting homepages, keywords and abstracts that are used to build indexes and directories that can be searched. Search sites use both indexes and directories (sometimes called search engines) to manage Internet information.

Web indexes are massive, computer-generated databases containing specific information related to millions of Web pages and/or Usenet newsgroup articles. The key to understanding indexes is that they are totally a computer-based approach to collecting and categorizing information. These indexes are continually up-dated. They can be searched for the specific information you need. Classic Web Indexes are *AltaVista Search* (www.altavista.digital.com), *Hot-Bot* (www.hotbot.com), *Open Text Index* (index.opentext.net) and *World Wide Web Worm* (www.cs.colorado.edu/wwww).

Web directories are lists of Web sites linked by hypertext, and hierarchically organized into categories by topic and subtopic. People, not just computers, create Web directories. Web directories often contain reviews or recommendations of sites. Because they are maintained by people reviewing sites, Web directories cover fewer sites, but the quality of information is often better targeted. Web directories can also be searched. *Yahoo!* (www.yahoo.com) and *Magellan Internet Guide* (www.mckinley.com) are primarily directories. *Excite* (www.excite.com), *Infoseek* (www.infoseek.com), *Lycos* (www.lycos.com) and *WebCrawler* (www.webcrawler.com) are hybrids, that offer both heavy-duty Web indexes and Web directories.

If you know the specific topic that you want to find, then you can use a keyword search through one of the indexes or hybrids. (See Figures 6.4 and 6.5 for an example).

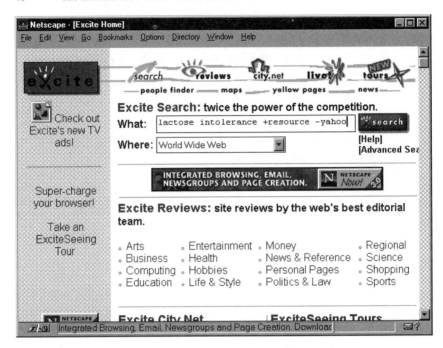

Figure 6.4 Initiating a Search using *Excite*

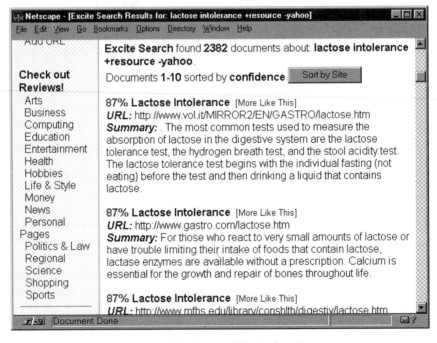

Figure 6.5 Results of *Excite* Search

However, if you're not looking for a specific piece of information, but rather want to browse a topic area, then a directory will allow you to drill down through sub-directories to narrow your search. (See Figures 6.6 through 6.8 for an example)

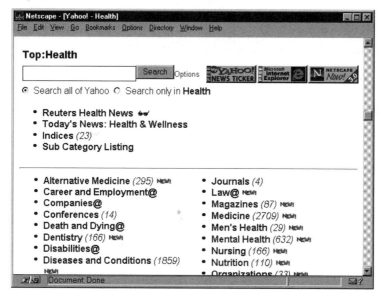

Figure 6.6 *Yahoo!* Health Directory

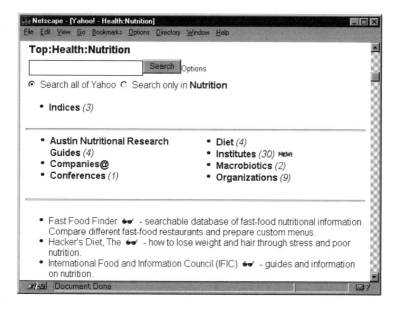

Figure 6.7 *Yahoo!* Health Subtopics

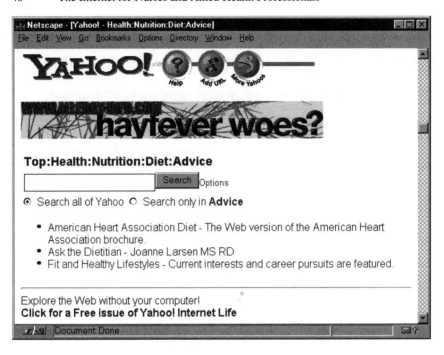

Figure 6.8 *Yahoo!* Health/Nutrition/Diet/Advice Subtopics

When you want the most comprehensive search possible, you can use a Metasearch site. Metasearch sites load your query (keyword search) simultaneously into many different indexes and directories. MetaCrawler (www. metacrawler.com), for example, simultaneously submits your search to nine different search engines.

There is no BEST search site or approach because your needs vary each time you want to find information on the Internet. In the examples above, it is very efficient to use a search site to locate very specific material related to lactose intolerance. However, if you just want to see what the Internet has to offer in an area such as nutrition, it may be much more profitable and efficient to use a directory and follow the links, or consult a catalogue such as the one provided in Appendix II.

If using the Web is so easy with a Web browser and search sites, why would you ever use Archie & friends or Gopher? As we noted at the beginning of the chapter, the key is to use the right tool for the job. Although you can use the Web to read Usenet articles, you are usually better off with a newsreader. You might first identify the newsgroup while browsing the Web, but a newsreader will then let you read articles from that newsgroup in a timely fashion. A second reason for using other retrieval systems is that not all information that you might be seeking is on the Web. A human somewhere has to put all the links in place for any one document. Multiply that times the number of documents that are available on the Internet and you have an enormous task. Taking into account that Web access only became widely available in 1993, you'll realize that many documents are still without Web links. Those documents can be accessed through the search system appropriate to the type of information you are seeking: Archie for FTP sites, Veronica or Jughead for Gopher sites and Wais for Wais sources. As the Web and browsers become more sophisticated, the need for Archie and friends will decrease. The documents that they search are becoming accessible through the Web and so are now appearing in Web indexes and directories.

Final Thoughts

As the Internet grows in popularity and its use becomes more a part of our lives, you can expect to see more tools developed to make it easier to locate the valuable information that is out there on the Net. In the meantime, the tools described in this chapter will help you discover the power and value of the Net.

7
Using and Citing Information from the Internet

Using Information from the Internet

The Internet is a wide-open frontier. Anyone can, for the cost of a homepage, put any type of information on the Internet. Therefore, a note of caution is necessary. All information on the Internet is not created equal. You must use your judgment in determining the validity and reliability of information that you find on the Internet. Sites that are moderated or sponsored by educational institutions, national/international associations or governments tend to provide more credible information. However, there are also some excellent personal sites, so your discernment is the key to using only credible information. If a site asks you to pay to see the information it provides, this should sound a cautionary note. Certainly you will have to pay to subscribe to services such as database searching through MEDLINE or CINAHL Direct, but a subscription such as this differs from the cybersnake oil that awaits the unwary.

Citing Information from the Internet

Intellectual property laws apply to all Internet materials including audio, video, graphics and text. It is necessary to cite Internet sources used in your research and writing just as you cite conventional print-based sources. Limited excerpts from the guidelines for citing information from the Internet according to APA and MLA style are reproduced here with the permission of the authors. For a more complete guide, see Li, X., & Crane, N.B. (1996). *Electronic Styles: A Handbook for Citing Electronic Information*, 2nd edition. Medford, NJ: Information Today. Updates to these guidelines can be found at **http://www.uvm. edu/~xli/reference/estyles.html**

Electronic Sources: APA Style of Citation

>>>Individual Works<<<

Basic forms, commercial supplier, and using an Internet protocol:

Author/editor. (Year). *Title* (edition), [Type of medium]. Producer (optional). Available: Supplier/Database identifier or number [Access date].
Author/editor. (Year). *Title* (edition), [Type of medium]. Producer (optional). Available Protocol (if applicable): Site/Path/File [Access date].

Examples:

* *Oxford English dictionary computer file:* On compact disc (2nd ed.), [CD-ROM]. (1992). Available: Oxford UP [1995, May 27].
* Pritzker, T. J. (No date). *An Early fragment from central Nepal* [Online]. Available:
http://www.ingress.com/~astanart/pritzker/pritzker.html [1995, June 8].
* Write "No date" when the electronic publication date is not available.
* When citing information retrieved on the World Wide Web, it is not necessary to repeat the protocol (HTTP) after "Available" since that
is stated in the URL.

>>>Parts of Works<<<

Basic forms, commercial supplier, and using an Internet protocol:

Author/editor. (Year). Title. In *Source* (edition), [Type of medium]. Producer (optional). Available: Supplier/Database identifier or number [Access date].
Author/editor. (Year). Title. In *Source* (edition), [Type of medium]. Producer (optional). Available Protocol (if applicable): Site/Path/File [Access date].

Examples:

* Bosnia and Hercegovina. (1995). In *Academic American Encyclopedia* [Online]. Available: Dow Jones News Retrieval Service/ENCYC [1995, June 5].
* This is an article from an encyclopedia with no author given.
* Daniel, R. T. (1995). The history of Western music. *In Britannica online: Macropaedia* [Online]. Available:
http://www.eb.com:180/cgi-bin/g:DocF=macro/5004/45/0.html [1995, June 14].

* When citing information retrieved on the World Wide Web, it is not necessary to repeat the protocol (HTTP) after "Available" since that
is stated in the URL.

>>>Journal Articles<<<

Basic forms, commercial supplier, and using an Internet protocol:

Author. (Year). Title. *Journal Title* [Type of medium], *volume*(issue),
paging or indicator of length. Available: Supplier/Database name
(Database identifier or number, if available)/Item or accession number
[Access date].
Author. (Year). Title. *Journal Title* [Type of medium], *volume*(issue),
paging or indicator of length. Available Protocol (if applicable):
Site/Path/File [Access date].

Examples:

* Clark, J. K. Complications in academia: Sexual harassment and the law.
Siecus Report [CD-ROM], 21(6), 6-10. Available: 1994 SIRS/SIRS 1993
School/Volume 4/Article 93A [1995, June 13].
* Carriveau, K. L., Jr. [Review of the book *Environmental hazards:*
Marine pollution]. *Electronic Green Journal* [Online], 2(1), 3
paragraphs. Available:
gopher://gopher.uidaho.edu/11/UI_gopher/library/egj03/carriv01.html
[1995, June 21].
* This is a reference for a book review; brackets indicate title is supplied.
* When citing information retrieved on the World Wide Web, it is not necessary to repeat the protocol (Gopher) after "Available" since that
is stated in the URL.
* Inada, K. (1995). A Buddhist response to the nature of human rights.
Journal of Buddhist Ethics [Online], 2, 9 paragraphs. Available:
http://www.cac.psu.edu/jbe/twocont.html [1995, June 21].
* When citing information retrieved on the World Wide Web, it is not necessary to repeat the protocol (HTTP) after "Available" since that
is stated in the URL.

>>>Magazine Articles<<<

Basic forms, commercial supplier, and using an Internet protocol:

Author. (Year, month day). Title. *Magazine Title* [Type of medium],
volume (if given), paging or indicator of length. Available:
Supplier/Database name (Database identifier or number, if

available)/Item or accession number [Access date].
Author. (Year, month day). Title. *Magazine Title* [Type of medium],
volume (if given), paging or indicator of length. Available Protocol
(if applicable): Site/Path/File [Access date].

Examples:

* Goodstein, C. (1991, September). Healers from the deep. *American Health*
[CD-ROM], 60-64. Available: 1994 SIRS/SIRS 1992 Life Science/Article 08A
[1995, June 13].
* Viviano, F. (1995, May/June0. The new Mafia order. *Mother Jones Magazine* [Online], 72 paragraphs. Available:
    http://www.mojones.com/MOTHER_JONES/MJ95/viviano.html [1995, July
17].
* When citing information retrieved on the World Wide Web, it is not necessary to repeat the protocol (HTTP) after "Available" since that is stated in the URL.

>>>Newspaper Articles<<<

Basic forms, commercial supplier, and using an Internet protocol:

Author. (Year, month day). Title. *Newspaper Title* [Type of medium],
paging or indicator of length. Available: Supplier/Database name
(Database identifier or number, if available)/Item or accession number
[Access date].
Author. (Year, month day). Title. *Newspaper Title* [Type of medium],
paging or indicator of length. Available Protocol (if applicable):
Site/Path/File [Access date].

Examples:

* Howell, V., & Carlton, B. (1993, August 29). Growing up tough: New generation fights for its life: Inner-city youths live by rule of
    vengeance. *Birmingham News* [CD-ROM], p. 1A(10 pp.). Available: 1994
    SIRS/SIRS 1993 Youth/Volume 4/Article 56A [1995, July 16].
* Johnson, T. (1994, December 5). Indigenous people are now more combative, organized. *Miami Herald* [Online], p. 29SA(22
    paragraphs).Available: gopher://summit.fiu.edu/Miami
    Herald--Summit-Related Articles/12/05/95--Indigenous People Now More
    Combative, Organized [1995, July 16].
* This reference gives beginning page and the number of paragraphs; this information is useful if one wishes to refer to material in text
    references.

* When citing information retrieved on the World Wide Web, it is not necessary to repeat the protocol (HTTP) after "Available" since that
is stated in the URL.

>>>Discussion List Messages<<<

Basic forms:

> Author. (Year, Month day). Subject of message. *Discussion List* [Type
> of medium]. Available E-mail: DISCUSSION LIST@e-mail address
> [Access date].
> Author. (Year, Month day). Subject of message. *Discussion List* [Type
> of medium]. Available E-mail: LISTSERV@e-mail address/Get [Access
> date].

Examples:

> * RRECOME. (1995, April 1). Top ten rules of film criticism. *Discussions on
> All Forms of Cinema* [Online]. Available E-mail:
> CINEMA-L@american.edu [1995, April 1].
> * Author's login name, in uppercase, is given as the first element.

> Discussions on All Forms of Cinema [Online]. Available E-mail:
> LISTSERV@american.edu/Get cinema-l log9504A [1995, August 1].
> * Reference is obtained by searching the list's archive.

>>>Personal Electronic Communications (E-mail)<<<

Basic forms:

> Sender (Sender's E-mail address). (Year, Month day). Subject of
> Message. E-mail to recipient (Recipient's E-mail address)

Examples:

> * Day, Martha (MDAY@sage.uvm.edu). (1995, July 30). Review of film—
> *Bad Lieutenant*. E-mail to Xia Li (XLI@moose.uvm.edu).

Electronic Sources: MLA Style of Citation

>>>Individual Works<<<

Basic forms, commercial supplier, and using an Internet protocol:

Author/editor. *Title of Print Version of Work.* Edition statement (if given). Place of publication: publisher, date. *Title of Electronic Work.* Medium. Information supplier. File identifier or number. Access date.

Author/editor. *Title of Print Version of Work.* Edition statement (if given). Publication information (Place of publication: publisher, date), if given. *Title of Electronic Work.* Medium. Information supplier. Available Protocol (if applicable): Site/Path/File. Access date.

Examples:

* *Oxford English Dictionary Computer File: On Compact Disc.* 2nd ed. CD-ROM. Oxford: Oxford UP, 1992.
* Pritzker, Thomas J. *An Early Fragment from Central Nepal.* N.D. Online. Ingress Communications. Available: http://www.ingress.com/~astanart/pritzker/pritzker.html. 8 June 1995.
* This is a citation form when the print version is not included in the reference.
* When citing information retrieved on the World Wide Web, it is not necessary to repeat the protocol (HTTP) after "Available" since that is stated in the URL.

>>>Parts of Works<<<

Basic forms, commercial supplier, and using an Internet protocol:

Author/editor. "Part title." *Title of Print Version of Work.* Edition statement (if given). Place of publication: publisher, date. *Title of Electronic Work.* Medium. Information supplier. File identifier or number. Access date.

Author/editor. "Part title." *Title of Print Version of Work.* Edition statement (if given). Publication information (Place of publication: publisher, date), if given. *Title of Electronic Work.* Medium. Information supplier. Available Protocol (if applicable): Site/Path/File. Access date.

Examples:

* "Bosnia and Hercegovina." *Academic American Encyclopedia.* 1995.
Academic American Encyclopedia. Online. Dow Jones News Retrieval
Service. ENCYC. 5 June 1995.
* This is an article from an encyclopedia with no author given.
* It is not necessary to give place of publication and publisher when citing
well-known reference sources.
* Daniel, Ralph Thomas. "The History of Western Music." *Britannica Online:*
Macropaedia. 1995. Online. Encyclopedia Britannica. Available:
http://www.eb.com:180/cgi-bin/g:DocF=macro/5004/45/0.html. 14 June
1995.
* It is not necessary to give place of publication and publisher when citing
well-known reference sources.
* When citing information retrieved on the World Wide Web, it is not necessary to repeat the protocol (HTTP) after "Available" since that
is stated in the URL.

>>>Journal Articles<<<

Basic forms, commercial supplier, and using an Internet protocol:

Author. "Article Title." *Journal Title.* Volume.Issue (Year): paging or
indicator or length. Medium. Information supplier. *Database Name.* File
identifier or number. Accession number. Access date.
Author. "Article Title." *Journal Title.* Volume.Issue (Year): paging or
indicator or length. Medium. Available Protocol (if applicable):
Site/Path/File. Access date.

Examples:

* Clark, Jeffrey K. "Complications in Academia: Sexual Harassment and the
Law." *Siecus Report.* 21.6 (1993): 6-10. CD-ROM. 1994 SIRS. *SIRS*
1993 School. Volume 4. Article 93A.
* Access date is not needed when the medium is a CD-ROM.
* Carriveau, Kenneth L., Jr. Rev. of *Environmental Hazards: Marine Pollu-*
tion, by Marth Gonnan. *Environmental Green Journal* 2.1 (1995): 3
pars. Online. Available:
gopher://gopher.uidaho.edu/11/UI_gopher/library/egj03/carriv01.html.
21 June 1995.
* This is a reference for a book review.
* For paging information, substitute number of paragraphs, i.e., "3 pars." for
three paragraphs in this reference.
* When citing information retrieved on the World Wide Web, it is not necessary to repeat the protocol (Gopher) after "Available" since that

is stated in the URL.

* Inada, Kenneth. "A Buddhist Response to the Nature of Human Rights." *Journal of Buddhist Ethics 2* (1995): 9 pars. Online. Available: http://www.cac.psu.edu/jbe/twocont.html. 21 June 1995.

* When citing information retrieved on the World Wide Web, it is not necessary to repeat the protocol (HTTP) after "Available" since that
is stated in the URL.

>>>Magazine Articles<<<

Basic forms, commercial supplier, and using an Internet protocol:

Author. "Article Title." *Magazine Title*. Date: paging or indicator or length. Medium. Information supplier. *Database Name*. File identifier or number. Accession number. Access date.
Author. "Article Title." *Magazine Title*. Date: paging or indicator or length. Medium. Available Protocol (if applicable): Site/Path/File. Access date.

Examples:

* Goodstein, Carol. "Healers from the Deep." *American Health*. Sept. 1991: 60-64. CD-ROM. 1994 SIRS. *SIRS 1992 Life Science*. Article 08A.
* Access date is not needed when the medium is a CD-ROM.
* Viviano, Frank. "The New Mafia Order." *Mother Jones Magazine* May-June 1995: 72 pars. Online. Available:
http://www.mojones.com/MOTHER_JONES/MJ95/viviano.html.
17 July 1995.
* When citing information retrieved on the World Wide Web, it is not necessary to repeat the protocol (HTTP) after "Available" since that
is stated in the URL.

>>>Newspaper Articles<<<

Basic forms, commercial supplier, and using an Internet protocol:

Author. "Article Title." Newspaper Title. Date, Edition (if given): paging or indicator or length. Medium. Information supplier. *Database Name*. File identifier or number. Accession number. Access date.
Author. "Article Title." *Newspaper Title*. Date, Edition (if given): paging or indicator or length. Medium. Available Protocol (if applicable): Site/Path/File. Access date.

Examples:

* Howell, Vicki, and Bob Carlton. "Growing up Tough: New Generation Fights for Its Life: Inner-city Youths Live by Rule of Vengeance."
 Birmingham News. 29 Aug. 1993: 1A+. CD-ROM. 1994 SIRS. *SIRS 1993 Youth*. Volume 4. Article 56A.
 * Access date is not needed when the medium is a CD-ROM.
 * Johnson, Tim. "Indigenous People Are Now More Combative, Organized."
 Miami Herald 5 Dec. 1994: 29SA. Online. Available:
 gopher://summit.fiu.edu/Miami Herald--Summit-Related
 Articles/12/05/95--Indigenous People Now More Combative, Organized. 16 July 1995. 17 July 1995.
 * When citing information retrieved on the World Wide Web, it is not necessary to repeat the protocol (Gopher) after "Available" since that
 is stated in the URL.

>>>Discussion List Messages<<<

Basic forms:

 Author. "Subject of Message." Date. Online posting. Discussion List.
 Available E-mail: DISCUSSION LIST@e-mail address. Access date.
 Author. "Subject of Message." Date. Online posting. Discussion List.
 Available E-mail: LISTSERV@e-mail address/Get. Access date.

Examples:

* RRECOME. "Top Ten Rules of Film Criticism." 1 Apr. 1995. Online posting. Discussions on All Forms of Cinema. Available E-mail:
 CINEMA-L@american.edu. 1 Apr. 1995.
 * Author's login name, in uppercase, is given as the first element.
 * RRECOME. "Top Ten Rules of Film Criticism." 1 Apr. 1995. Online posting. Discussions on All Forms of Cinema. Available E-mail:
 LISTSERV@american.edu/Get cinema-l log9504A. 1 Aug. 1995.
 * Reference is obtained by searching the list's archive.

>>>Personal electronic communications (E-mail)<<<

Basic forms:

 Sender (Sender's E-mail address). "Subject of Message." E-mail to recipient (Recipient's E-mail address). Date of message.

Examples:

> * Day, Martha (MDAY@sage.uvm.edu). "Review of film—*Bad Lieutenant*."
> E-mail to Xia Li (XLI@moose.uvm.edu). 30 July 1995.

8
Implications for the Future: Science Fiction Versus Reality

Richard S. Hannah Ph.D

The Internet as we know it today is no longer exclusively a university-based network. Various commercial networks and enterprises now comprise the majority of sites available on the Net. In order to assess the future impact we must consider the implications of a true information superhighway. It is still pretty much a mystery as to what the evolving information superhighway will look like even in two years time. Will the Internet form the backbone or will it be absorbed into a larger amalgamation involving cable television systems, telephone companies, governments, computer manufacturing and software companies? We would really have to be card carrying Luddites to assume that some type of all-encompassing information superhighway will not be a reality before the turn of the century. After all, automobiles were never going to replace horses, steam would never replace sails and television was a flash in the pan!

No matter what form the Internet may take in the future, it is fair to say that everything developed for and available on a computer, will be accessible via the Internet.

Variables

The potential for real advances in the near term for health care on the Internet is predicated on the following conditions occurring:
1. Continuation of the rapid increase in computer purchases amongst health care practitioners and a demonstrable demand to professional societies, universities, hospitals and commercial vendors from current and potential users for more services. The major limitation to Net use is still the affordability factor. Unless you are lucky enough to have free access to a computer you are looking at around 3 to 4 thousand dollars just to get started. In the very near future we will see the arrival of cut down or Network only computers which will consist of little more than a keyboard/mouse and a monitor. Recent studies have demonstrated that most computer owners only make use of 20% of available features. You will not

need a hard drive because the server or large computer that you log on to will give you access to all of the software and features you will ever require, for a fee of course. This is referred to as the "sandbox" server. In other words, you pay to play in a commercial sandbox where all of the toys belong to the company and you just pay for those that you use. This will mean that you will not be faced with buying software which rapidly becomes obsolete, you merely rent it for a few minutes. Of course, this means you will need very little in the way of initial capital outlay for either hardware or software. In fact, one could easily envisage a smart black box along the lines of the one that you already rent from your cable company to access pay for view movies which will provide Net access using the TV set as the monitor. This type of economical service would also be a major breakthrough in delivering information to and dialoging with patients in their homes regardless of their socio-economic status.

2. If I may be philosophical, the biggest factor to consider when contemplating the future of health information via the Internet is human nature. Are we genuinely ready to make the leap to a paperless environment in our professional or for that matter our personal lives? Let's look at the example of electronic mail. Many of our colleagues still make manual drafts of all correspondence. When composing replies or new messages over a few lines in length, they write it out using good old pen and paper (probably fountain pen) and then have someone else enter it into the computer! Can we adapt our information gathering and learning skills to downplay the need to see it on paper? Since humanity first set pen to papyrus, we have had this innate (perhaps genetically coded) belief that unless it is on paper we just don't feel comfortable. It will certainly not be a quick evolution, our guess is at least a decade must pass before we quit treating hard copy as a psychological crutch.

3. One of the most pressing and serious decisions required in the near future, which will impact on the availability of learning material on the Internet, is copyright protection. If the material is on the Internet, it can easily be removed, copied and utilized without reference or compensation to the creators or originators. There are many sites on the Internet today that provide free access to a variety of computer-assisted instruction programs and health-related data. However, you will find that most of these sites only provide demonstrations of their material and not complete substantive packages. The obvious reason for this occurrence is, of course, that only the truly naive or philanthropic author is prepared to place his creations on-line in the absence of any controls to protect intellectual property. Medical illustrators, for example, represent a particularly vulnerable group. Certainly, piracy has occurred in the past with unscrupulous individuals using photography or the ubiquitous copying machine. Until Internet access to material became available, it was only well equipped facilities with high cost scanning equipment that could "borrow" material from hard copy publications and reproduce it on the computer. However, when presented with unlimited

digital images, animations and video clips, seemingly for the taking, there is a great temptation to borrow without permission or royalty payment. Perhaps one solution would be to establish consortia under the auspices of professional societies or universities. Access would be restricted to those individuals willing to sign a copyright acknowledgment for free use. Alternately, a contributor could be paid a royalty on a per use basis from a society that underwrites the cost from subscriptions or general dues. Then and only then will we see an explosion of commercial quality material on the Internet. That is not to say that commercial enterprises may not also undertake the provision of similar services. It is one thing to photocopy an entire book, but once the material appears on your computer screen there is no control over illegal copies that are virtually free.

4.   With the dramatic increase of health information appearing on the Net there comes with it the inherent problem of information quality. Whether you are a health professional or a consumer of health information you will be faced with judging the validity of the information. The health information explosion is happening so fast that the professional societies are scrambling to establish guidelines for content providers. With the ever present specter of censorship hovering in the background, where will we draw the line in offering a "Seal of Approval". Will this mean authorized or officially sanctioned sites where the motto is "9 out of 10 professionals use our site"? After all, products from toothpaste to toilet tissue claim sanctioning by one professional body or another. The appearance of standards in some form will be with us in the near future, let's hope that they are not so restrictive that they suppress new ideas.

Impact of the Internet on Health Care

Education programs

Electronic books

Is the age of the hard copy text book or journal dead or at least in its last death throes? Some book publishers are currently bringing out their line of text books on CD ROM and more appear every month. Since the textual material and some of the pictures already live on their own computer systems, it is fairly inexpensive for them to make the switch. However, the really exciting developments will come when the authors have opportunity to embellish their existing and future works with video clips, animations, audio explanations, etc. What appears to be holding them back are market surveys that show that very few people as yet have CD ROM players, so where would the profit be? First of all, a large percentage of the cost for paper books is the printing and transportation (50-60%), certainly not royalties to the authors! By going to CD-ROM, the profit margin rises dramatically! Hopefully they will soon figure out that the current small numbers of CD-ROM players can be overcome by putting the book on the Internet. New editions would occur much more frequently because the publishers would no longer be faced with what they are going to do with a warehouse full of unsold paper or for that matter CD-ROM editions. Publishers could establish an annual fee for each "textbook". Instead of going to the book shop and buying the hard copy or CD-ROM, you could purchase access to the whole book for varying time periods or maybe just the bits and pieces you need.

Simulations of Clinical Situations

Computer simulations are truly the wave of the future. During the next few years we can expect to see increasing numbers of simulations designed to carry us into a clinical situation with three dimensional images, sound and yes, even touch. For example, you are a physiotherapy student and a patient "arrives" on your computer screen and complains about a sore knee. You will be able to ask the patient questions, examine, test, diagnose the problem and treat the knee!

Continuing Education

For many health care practitioners, continuing education is a daunting and usually expensive task when faced with taking time off work and traveling to a central site. We can look forward to many or all of the professional societies and universities offering a wide range of specialty courses and credit programs via the Internet. The result would be similar to doing a correspondence course by mail, except that lessons would contain sound, video, animations and feedback from the instructor. It also would be available 24 hours a day 7 days a week from the privacy of your home or workplace. Thanks to the Internet, it also will be possible to take accredited courses at a wide variety of institutions around the world! How about signing up for a refresher course on temporal-mandibular joint pain, taught by an internationally recognized authority, being offered from a university on the other side of the world?

Distance Education

Perhaps distance education via the Internet will provide the mechanism for educational institutions to give serious thought to the problem of finding enough tax dollars to build new edifices of concrete and glass. The rapidly increasing numbers of multimedia educational programs will soon result in portions of courses, complete courses and even entire curricula being delivered and "consumed" in the home. Obviously, there will still be a need in some areas, to assemble as a group, but these situations will represent only a small proportion of the total instructional time.

Personal Communication

Some of the potential benefits of increased personal communication, nationally and internationally that can be achieved via e-mail and list servers are as follows:

1. *Practice standards* — participation in a world wide forum on those matters that affect our professions. Many societies only meet once or twice a year and we all know that the business meeting that inevitably occurs at the close of the conference attracts but a handful of members.
2. *Remuneration equity* — Are you being paid fairly? Discuss it at your next virtual class reunion on the Net.
3. *Sharing of old and new treatment methods*- Try out some of your ideas on your colleagues
4. *Training programs* — How does my program fare when compared with the rest of the world?
5. *Advice* — on all matters ranging from "How do I do this?" to "Have you ever seen this before?" then receive counsel from a pool of thousands of peers.

Information Gathering

Libraries around the world are already supplying services such as general access to their holdings. There are also a few that will mail (e-mail of course) you the table of contents and abstracts of your favorite journals when each new edition is received. What about the future? I think that the day of the paper journal is almost over. It will not be long before most of the scientific journals will be available electronically; initially on CD-ROMs. Libraries will most likely allow access to these electronic journals to their subscribers, over the Internet. This is already being done in one form using databases such as "Silver Platter". There are a number of on-line journals listed in Appendix II.

Databases ranging in content from dental x-ray libraries to pharmaceutical prices are already accessible to a special few on the Internet. We can look forward to an easing of access restrictions and a logarithmic increase in the quantity and variety of databases available for our perusal. You could even create your own database to store your data (such as x-rays or patient records). For example, why be confronted with the cost of buying and maintaining large storage devices such as hard drives or optical drives? Why not buy some space at a commercial enterprise or go together with some colleagues either locally, nationally or internationally and store your records electronically in a central location? Yes, shop around, you may find it cheaper to store your information two continents and 8 time zones away. After all, on the Internet, distance is not a factor!

Decision Support

Decision support programs will provide instantaneous responses to your queries. Our ability to help patients is routinely hampered by a lack of information and knowledge at the time and place that we are required to make health care-related decisions. This global access will make it much easier to cope with these situations and greatly enhance our ability to help the patient. Let's suppose that we are presented with a difficult case that leaves us scratching our heads and the patient expects an answer now, not next week after we have contacted 10 other colleagues for help. By accessing our on-line decision support system, it will walk us through the situation. It will provide us with clues and other information that we had not thought of or had just plain forgotten and, voila, our problem is solved. The patient is helped and we have realized that we do not have to keep everything in our heads. We all need a little constructive help sometimes.

Telehealth

Imagine you are a nurse, probably working out of your home and office in the suburbs. You receive a call on your system from a client complaining of a fever and fits of coughing. You inspect the patient on the video link. Perhaps using some telemetry equipment such as a thermometer or stethoscope you instruct the patient to place the sensors on the appropriate places on her body and take the readings. You may suspect it is just a flu virus so you consult the local community health data base for flu strains going through the community and yes there it is. Same symptoms as you have just seen. You advise the patient that what she has is prevalent in the area now and not to worry. Oh yes let's not forget the time honored phrase "Take two aspirins and call me in the morning" for a follow up telexam! If on the other hand, the complaint was more serious and required tests not available as yet from home, the patient is referred to a central facility. Let's assume for the sake of argument that the attending physician doesn't have the expertise to make a diagnosis. The physician would then contact specialists, anywhere in the world, via the "system", transmit the results of diagnostic tests and have the patient examined long distance. By the same token many patients will be able to remain in their homes or be sent home from hospital earlier and have their vital signs monitored from a central facility. This will not only be more convenient and comfortable for the patient but it will make hospital administrators ecstatic. Similar scenarios can easily be imagined for all sectors of health care providers. This may sound very futuristic but there are currently, many pilot projects in the works attempting to achieve this result. In the commercial sector, there are many companies competing for our business to enable us to store and transmit everything from x-ray images to pathology slide images.

Health Education for the Public

What will access to the Net mean to the general public in terms of health care? One of the newest topics to blossom on the Web is the area of Consumer Health Informatics. It is within this area that we will see the greatest changes. As universal access becomes the norm instead of the exception, more and more patients, their families and interested consumers will seek out their own answers to their questions rather than arranging direct contact with the health profession. Electronic discussion groups on diverse topics such as brain tumors, lupus and breast cancer are beginning to appear where interested parties can share experiences, information, support and advice. This will mean that for any one topic, thousands of people world wide will be scouring the net for new information. How will the health professional of the near future react to patients and family members who arrive in the office with much more information on current treatments than practitioners themselves are aware of? A pragmatic person will not feel threatened but rather treat this phenomenon as a large unpaid volunteer workforce of literature reviewers.

Long Term Care Facilities

Several long term care facilities are currently providing Internet access to residents. In addition to providing a whole new world of information and entertainment, residents can actively participate in newsgroup debates ranging from hobbies to castigating or offering helpful advice to their elected members of government. I know of one case where a son, living in Cape Town, South Africa, keeps in touch daily with his elderly father who lives in a care facility in Toronto, Canada. Surprisingly, he "talks" to his father more now than he did when he lived in the same city. This is a simply marvelous idea that more institutions should adopt.

Conclusion (or Beginning?)

Bringing health care to the information superhighway will certainly be a multibillion dollar business. However, who will monitor the quality? Will it be the commercial sector that is probably going to fund most of it in the expectation of reaping great profits? Or will it be the government sector that doesn't have the money but would like the control? Or will it be the health care practitioners themselves? One can only hope that it will be a tripartite arrangement.

Regardless of who sets the stage, it seems clear that an information superhighway will greatly affect the practice of health care professionals. It is timely then for each professional to become aware of and proficient in the developing technology. Only then can you take advantage of what's available today and be in a position to develop the resources of tomorrow.

Appendix 1
Top Ten Favourite Web Sites

1. Food and Nutrition Information Center

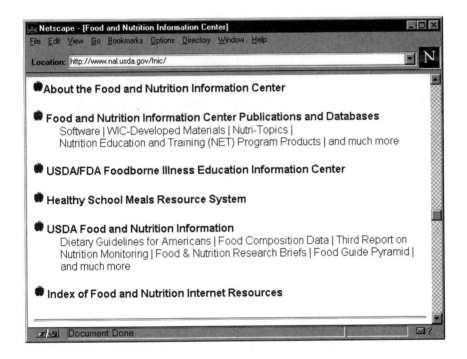

2. GoldenAge Net

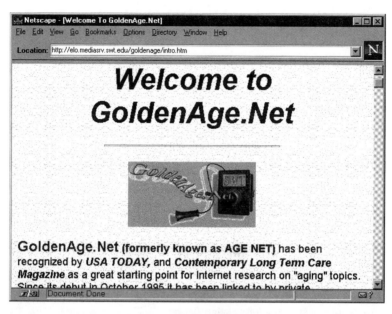

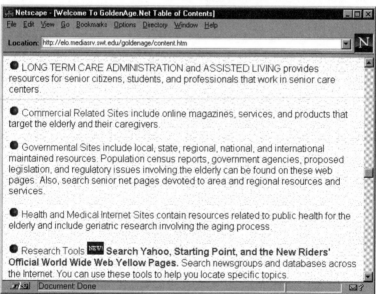

3. Hardin Meta Directory of Internet Health Sources

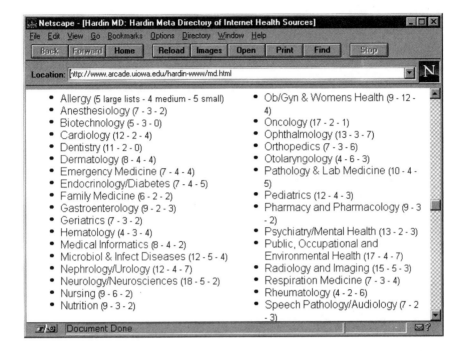

Netscape - [Hardin MD: Hardin Meta Directory of Internet Health Sources]

File   Edit   View   Go   Bookmarks   Options   Directory   Window   Help

Back   Forward   Home   Reload   Images   Open   Print   Find   Stop

Location: http://www.arcade.uiowa.edu/hardin-www/md.html

- Allergy (5 large lists - 4 medium - 5 small)
- Anesthesiology (7 - 3 - 2)
- Biotechnology (5 - 3 - 0)
- Cardiology (12 - 2 - 4)
- Dentistry (11 - 2 - 0)
- Dermatology (8 - 4 - 4)
- Emergency Medicine (7 - 4 - 4)
- Endocrinology/Diabetes (7 - 4 - 5)
- Family Medicine (6 - 2 - 2)
- Gastroenterology (9 - 2 - 3)
- Geriatrics (7 - 3 - 2)
- Hematology (4 - 3 - 4)
- Medical Informatics (8 - 4 - 2)
- Microbiol & Infect Diseases (12 - 5 - 4)
- Nephrology/Urology (12 - 4 - 7)
- Neurology/Neurosciences (18 - 5 - 2)
- Nursing (9 - 6 - 2)
- Nutrition (9 - 3 - 2)

- Ob/Gyn & Womens Health (9 - 12 - 4)
- Oncology (17 - 2 - 1)
- Ophthalmology (13 - 3 - 7)
- Orthopedics (7 - 3 - 6)
- Otolaryngology (4 - 6 - 3)
- Pathology & Lab Medicine (10 - 4 - 5)
- Pediatrics (12 - 4 - 3)
- Pharmacy and Pharmacology (9 - 3 - 2)
- Psychiatry/Mental Health (13 - 2 - 3)
- Public, Occupational and Environmental Health (17 - 4 - 7)
- Radiology and Imaging (15 - 5 - 3)
- Respiration Medicine (7 - 3 - 4)
- Rheumatology (4 - 2 - 6)
- Speech Pathology/Audiology (7 - 2 - 3)

Document Done

4. Magellan: Health and Medicine

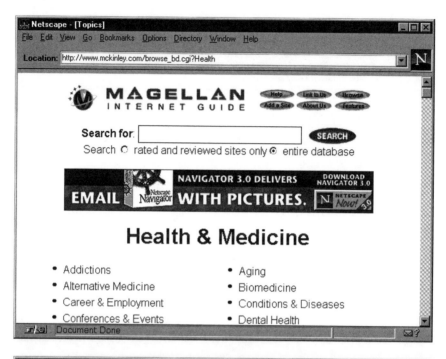

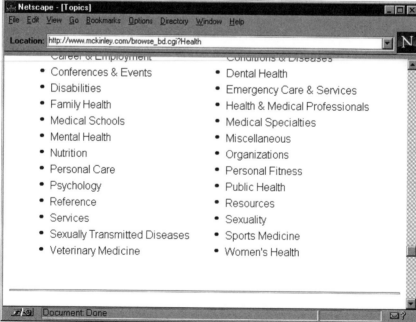

5. MedWeb

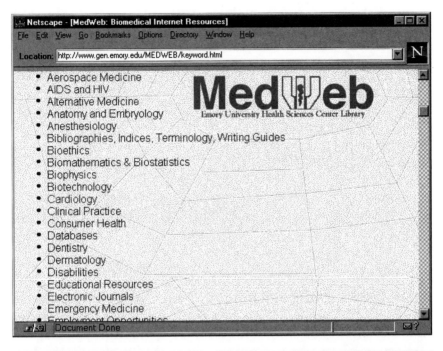

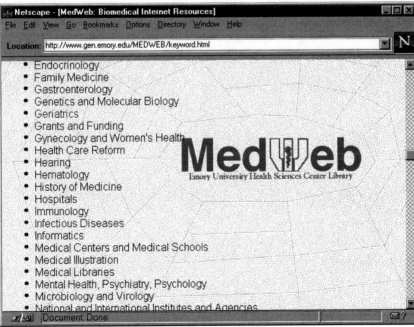

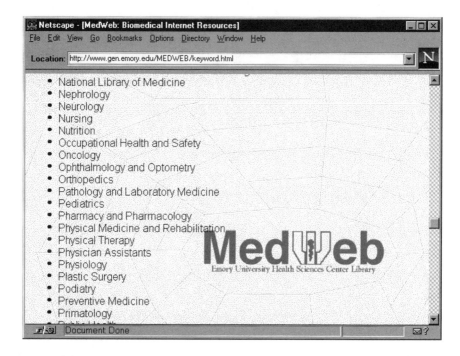

6. Peter Ramme's Idea Nurse

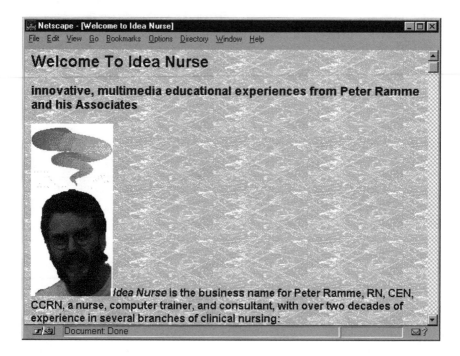

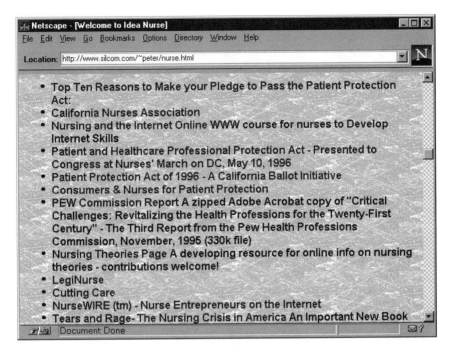

Netscape - [Welcome to Idea Nurse]

File Edit View Go Bookmarks Options Directory Window Help

Location: http://www.silcom.com/~peter/nurse.html

- Top Ten Reasons to Make your Pledge to Pass the Patient Protection Act:
- California Nurses Association
- Nursing and the Internet Online WWW course for nurses to Develop Internet Skills
- Patient and Healthcare Professional Protection Act - Presented to Congress at Nurses' March on DC, May 10, 1996
- Patient Protection Act of 1996 - A California Ballot Initiative
- Consumers & Nurses for Patient Protection
- PEW Commission Report A zipped Adobe Acrobat copy of "Critical Challenges: Revitalizing the Health Professions for the Twenty-First Century" - The Third Report from the Pew Health Professions Commission, November, 1995 (330k file)
- Nursing Theories Page A developing resource for online info on nursing theories - contributions welcome!
- LegiNurse
- Cutting Care
- NurseWIRE (tm) - Nurse Entrepreneurs on the Internet
- Tears and Rage- The Nursing Crisis in America An Important New Book

Document Done

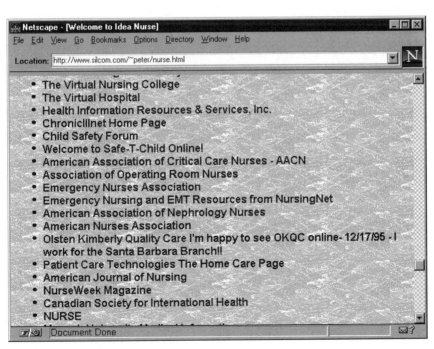

Netscape - [Welcome to Idea Nurse]

File Edit View Go Bookmarks Options Directory Window Help

Location: http://www.silcom.com/~peter/nurse.html

- The Virtual Nursing College
- The Virtual Hospital
- Health Information Resources & Services, Inc.
- ChronicIllnet Home Page
- Child Safety Forum
- Welcome to Safe-T-Child Online!
- American Association of Critical Care Nurses - AACN
- Association of Operating Room Nurses
- Emergency Nurses Association
- Emergency Nursing and EMT Resources from NursingNet
- American Association of Nephrology Nurses
- American Nurses Association
- Olsten Kimberly Quality Care I'm happy to see OKQC online- 12/17/95 - I work for the Santa Barbara Branch!!
- Patient Care Technologies The Home Care Page
- American Journal of Nursing
- NurseWeek Magazine
- Canadian Society for International Health
- NURSE

Document Done

7. Points of Interest: Pediatrics

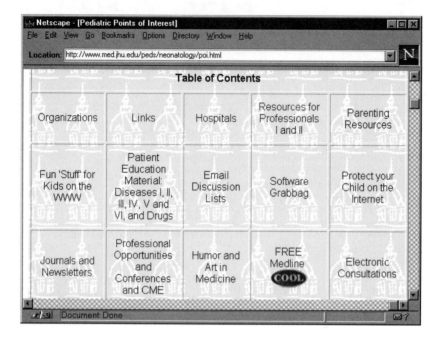

8. Virtual Hospital

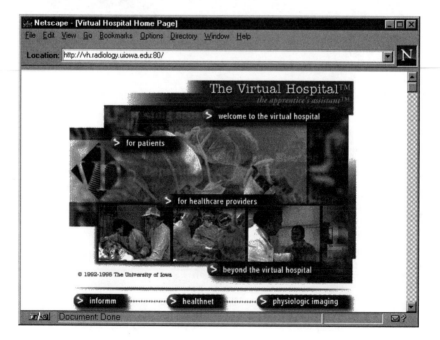

9. Virtual Pharmacy

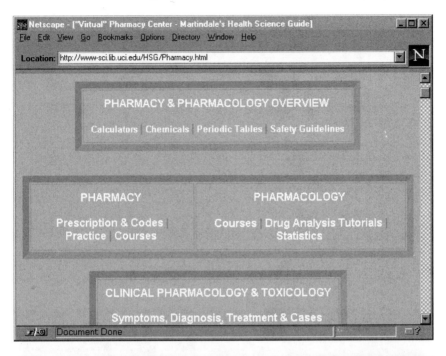

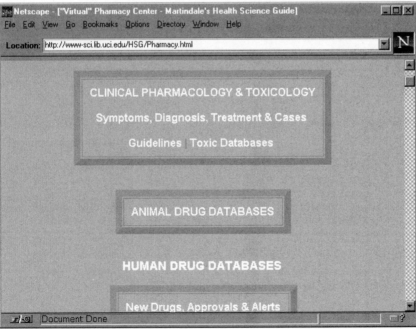

10. Yahoo! Health Directory

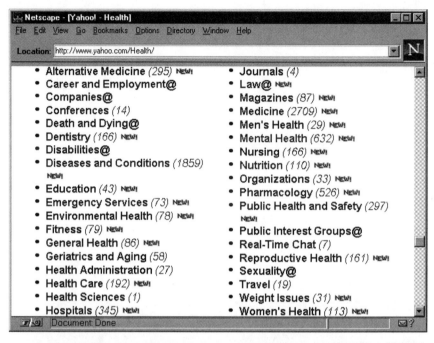

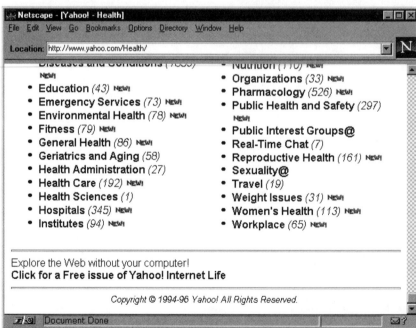

Appendix 2
Health-Related Internet Resources

Profession Specific

Nursing

Academic Journal Directory

Contains listings for over 400 professional academic journals related to clinical nursing, nursing education, research and related healthcare fields. Each listing includes journal name, publisher, frequency of publication, types of manuscripts it reviews and submission guidelines.

World Wide Web:
 URL: **http://129.109.57.215/catalog/catalog.htm**

American Journal of Nursing

Offers links to on-line versions of the current and previous editions and a pre-view of the next edition of American Journal of Nursing, The American Journal of Maternal/Child Nursing and Nursing Research. Also provides a con-nection to AJN Network (see below)

World Wide Web:
 URL: **http://www.ajn.org**

American Journal of Nursing Network

Offers forums on various areas of nursing including med-surg, Maternal-child, Psych-mental health, emergency, management, gerontology, rural nursing and home health and for various roles including educator, administrator, researcher, advanced practice, student and case manager. This site often takes a long time to connect, so be patient! It also offers databases of multimedia catalogues, nurse organizations, and upcoming conferences. Also offered are a Career center and peer consultation.

World Wide Web:
URL: **http://www.ajn.org/ajnnet**

Telnet:
Address: **ajn.org**
Login: **new**

American Nurses Association

World Wide Web:
URL: **http://www.nursingworld.org/ana.htm**

Galaxy Index of Nursing-related Services on the Internet

Provides extensive links to other nursing-related resources available on the Internet, including Nursing Research, Nursing Theory and Nursing Specialties. Also includes On-line Journal of Issues in Nursing, links to professional and academic organizations.

World Wide Web:
URL: **http://galaxy.einet.net/galaxy/Medicine/Nursing.html**

HEALTHWEB: NURSING

Provides information and links related to career information, clinical nursing, education. organizations, research and other resources.

World Wide Web:
URL: **http://www.lib.umich.edu/tml/nursing.html**

NIGHTINGALE

Offers many links/sub menus related to research, practice and education. The sub-menus of the specific sections are detailed below. Many of these are still under development. The Web page also offers information about upcoming conferences and calls for papers.

World Wide Web:
> URL: **http://nightingale.con.utk.edu:70/0/homepage.html**

Gopher:
> URL: **gopher://nightingale.con.utk.edu/1**
> **Research** sub-menu

Contains information about grants, abstracts, newsletters, communications about research groups' activities, a list of experts by area of expertise, research methodology articles and computer resources organized by topic.
> URL: **gopher://nightingale.con.utk.edu:70/11/Research**
> **Practice** sub-menu

Contains information about nursing policies at national, state and local levels, care plans, and diagnostic and measurement tools useful for the practicing nurse.
> URL: **gopher://nightingale.con.utk.edu:70/11/Practice**
> **Education** sub-menu

Provides information about many educational institutions around the world. This includes departmental information, course description and entrance requirements, and faculty and staff. Also included is information about education supplies, such as textbooks, CAI, software, videos and yellow pages for clinical skills teaching materials.
> URL: **gopher://nightingale.con.utk.edu:70/11/Education**
> **Professional nursing communications** sub-menu

Includes information about conferences, grants, computer discussion groups and announcements of job positions.
> URL: **gopher://nightingale.con.utk.edu:70/11/Communications**

Nursing and the NCLEX

Has links to information about the types of question, scoring and test plan of the NCLEX. Sample question from a variety of areas are also available. Also includes information related to selecting a graduate program and conducting a job search.

World Wide Web:
> URL: **http://www.kaplan.com:80/nclex/**

NURSE

Provides links to related directories, resource guides, gopher sites, newsgroups and mailing lists.

World Wide Web:
> URL: http://med714.bham.ac.uk/nursing/

Nurse Net Nederland

A Web site in the Netherlands that offers links to other nursing sites and also to a bulletin board service.

World Wide Web:
> URL: **http://care4all.nursing.nl:8080/index.html**

Nursing Network Forum on Delphi

Provides on-line continuing education for nurses. Also offered is a bulletin board service and a job search facility.

Telnet:
> Address: **delphi.com**
> Login: **joindelphi**
> Password: **custom**
> Referral name: **NURSE1**   (this entitles you to five free hours)
> at any prompt, type **GO CUS 261** to get to the Nursing Network Forum

Serveurs sur l'Internet dans le domain de la Sante

This site includes lists of health-related sites, electronic journals, searchable databases, such as Medline, and articles related to a variety of medical & nursing specialties, all in French.

World Wide Web:
> URL: http://www.chu.rouen.fr/ssm/watch.html

Peter Ramme's Idea Nurse

Offers links to innovative education opportunities for nurses. Links connect to on-line courses such as Other links are to other nursing related-resources on the Internet. This is an excellent place to look for nursing resources!

World Wide Web:
>   URL: **http://www.silcom.com/~peter/nurse.html**

WHO Nursing Bulletin Board

This site offers services in English, French and Spanish. In addition to links to other nursing sites, it provides reports of Study Groups and recent World Health Assembly Resolutions.

World Wide Web:
>   URL: **http://www.who.ch:80/programmes/nur/english.htm**
>   **http://www.who.ch:80/programmes/nur/francais.htm**
>   **http://www.who.ch:80/programmes/nur/espa_bbs.htm**

The "Virtual" Nursing Centre

Has links to nursing schools, courses and educational resources.

World Wide Web:
>   URL: **http://www.sci.lib.uci.edu:80/`martindale/Nursing.html**

Duke University School of Nursing

World Wide Web:
>   URL: **http://son3.mc.duke.edu/**

East Tennessee State University College of Nursing

World Wide Web:
>   URL: **http://www.etsu-tn.edu/etsucon/index.htm**

Ohio State University College of Nursing

World Wide Web:
>   URL: **http://www.con.ohio-state.edu:80/**

Texas A&M University-Corpus Christi-Department of Nursing and Health Sciences

World Wide Web:
　　URL: **http://www.sci.tamucc.edu/nursing**

University of California: San Francisco School of Nursing

World Wide Web:
　　URL: **http://nurseweb.ucsf.edu/www/son.htm**

University of Delaware School of Nursing

World Wide Web:
　　URL: **http://www.udel.edu/brentt/UD_Nursing.html**

University of Iowa School of Nursing

World Wide Web:
　　URL: **http://coninfo.nursing.UIOWA.EDU**

University of Maryland School of Nursing

World Wide Web:
　　URL: **http://www.nursing.ab.umd.edu/**

University of Pennsylvania School of Nursing

World Wide Web:
　　URL: **http://www.upenn.edu/overview/schools.html**

University of Washington School of Nursing

World Wide Web:
 URL: **http://www.son.hs.washington.edu/**

Virtual Nursing

Provides links to tutorials, including graphics, on chronic wound care and Cancer pain education for patients and families. Still under development, but looks interesting!

World Wide Web:
 URL: **http://coninfo.nursing.UIOWA.EDU/www/
 nursing/virtnurs/virtnurs.htm**

Listservers

CULTURE-AND-NURSING
 To join, send a message to **majordomo@itssrvll.ucsf.**edu with **subscribe CULTURE-AND-NURSING** in the body of the message

NURSENET
 To join, send mail to **LISTSERV@VM.UTCC.UTORONTO.CA.SUB NURSENET** with **subscribe NURSENET <first name> <last name>** in the body of the message.

GradNrse (Graduate Nurses List)
 To join send mail to **LISTSERV@KENTVM.KENT.EDU** with **SUB GradNrse <first-name> <last-name>** in the body of the message.

Ivtherapy-L (IV therapy nursing)
 To join send mail to **majordomo@netcom.com** with **subscribe ivtherapy-L <first-name> <last-name>** in the body of the message.

NRSING-L (Nursing Informatics List)
 To join send mail to **listproc@nic.umass.edu** with **SUB nrsing-l <first-name> <last-name>** in the body of the message.

NURSENET
 To join send mail to **listserv@listserv.utoronto.ca** with **sub nursenet <first-name> <last-name>** in the body of the message.

NURSERES (Nurses Research List)
> To join send mail to **LISTSERV@KENTVM.KENT.EDU** with **SUB NURSERES <first-name> <last-name>** in the body of the message.

NRSINGED (Nursing Educators List)
> To join send mail to **listserv@ulkyvm.louisville.edu** with **SUB NRSINGED <first-name> <last-name>** in the body of the message.

NURSE-UK (UK nursing issues)
> To join send mail to **nurse-uk-request@csv.warwick.ac.uk** with **sub-scribe NURSE-UK <first name> <last name>** in the body of the message.

QUALRS-L (Qualitative Research for the Human Sciences)
> To join send mail to **LISTSERV@UGA.CC.UGA.EDU** with **sub qualrs-l <first-name> <last-name>** in the body of the message.

Psychiatric-Nursing
> To join send mail to **mailbase@mailbase.ac.uk** with **subscribe Psychiatric-Nursing <first name> <last name>** in the body of the message.

SCHLRN-L (School nurse list)
> To join send mail to **LISTSERV@UBVM.CC.BUFFALO.EDU** with **SUB CHLRN-L <first name> <last name>** in the body of the message.

SNURS-L (For undergraduate nursing students)
> To join, send mail to **listserv@abvm.cc.buffalo.edu** with **SUB snurse-l <first name> <last name>** in the body of the message.

Newsgroups:

Usenet:
> newsgroup: **alt.npractitioners** (for nurse practitioners)
> newsgroup: **sci.med.nursing**
> newsgroup: **bit.listserv.snurse-l** (for student nurses)

Medical Laboratory Technology

Medical Laboratory Associations

Provides links to a variety of specialty-based associations.

World Wide Web:
URL: **http://www.ualberta.ca/~pletendre/medassoc.html**

Listservers

MEDLAB-L
To join send mail to **listserv@vm.ucs.ualberta.ca** with **subscribe MEDLAB-L <first name> <last name>** in the body of the message.

Nutrition

American Dietetics Association

Information for members, and about up-coming conferences.

World Wide Web:
URL: **http://www.plsgroup.com/dg/3d36.html**

American Institute of Nutrition

Information about the Institute, awards and competitions, publications and membership information.

World Wide Web:
URL: **http://www.faseb.org/ain**

Food Science and Technology at Cornell University

Provides links to information about its on-campus and distance education courses.

World Wide Web:
URL: **http://aruba.nysaes.cornell.edu**

University of Minnesota—Department of Food Science and Nutrition

Offers links to information about its programs, other network sites and Internet supported courses.

World Wide Web:
URL: **http://fscn1.fsci.umn.edu**

University of Wisconsin—River Falls Food Science and Technology

Provides links to information about its programs.

World Wide Web:
URL: **http://www.uwrf.edu/food-science/welcome.html**

Occupational Therapy

Occupational Therapy Links

A good list of links to a variety of occupational therapy associations, and resources.

World Wide Web:
URL: **http://www.rehabjob.com/links.htm**

Pharmacy

The "Virtual" Pharmacy Centre

Offers links to pharmacy schools, courses and educational resources.

World Wide Web:
URL: **http://www.sci.lib.uci.edu/HSG/Pharmacy.html**

Physician Assistants

The National PA Page

Provides links to information about physician assistants, undergraduate and graduate level educational programs, research, resource lists and job vacancy announcements.

World Wide Web:
  URL: **http://www.papage.com/papage/**

Physiotherapy

Charlie Kornberg's Physiotherapy Page

An interesting set of links to physio resources, conference announcements, full-text articles related to topics such as hamstrings and lumbar spine, tennis elbow, scoliosis, and cervicogenic headache.

World Wide Web:
  URL: **http://www.ozonline.com.au/physio**

HealthWeb: Physical Medicine/Physical Therapy

Evaluated resources for the physical medicine community includes links to specific associations and Centers, educational tools, and publications. A good beginning site for PT's

World Wide Web:
  URL: **http://hsinfo.ghsl.nwu.edu/healthweb/pmr/pt.html**

Physiotherapy Global-Links

An excellent site with journal articles and abstracts, research groups, schools & courses, conference announcements, job opportunities and links to mailing lists, newsgroups and other Web sites. Another good place to browse.

World Wide Web:
  URL: **http://www.netspot.unisa.edu.au/pt/index/html**

Listservers

PHYSIO
> To join send mail to **mailbase@mailbase.ac.uk** with **subscribe PHYSIO
> <first name> <last name>** in the body of the message.

Respiratory Therapy

Professional Associations

Links to international and national associations.

World Wide Web:
> URL: **http://www.cariboo.bc.ca/schs/aldhlth/i_sites.htm**

Respiratory Hot-Links

An extensive site providing on-line articles and links to other resources and sites related to specific disorders, employment, education and publications.

World Wide Web:
> URL: **http://www.xmission.com/~gastown/herpmed/respi.htm**

Newsgroups

Usenet:
> newsgroup: **bit.med.resp-care.world**

Health-related Topics

Addictions

Addiction Research Foundation

Offers public information materials related to a variety of topics including, alcohol, various recreational drugs, caffeine, and tobacco. Also has audiovisuals on above topics, links to other Net resources and a resource listing for health professionals.

World Wide Web:
   URL: **http://www.arf.org/isd/info.html**

Canadian Centre on Substance Abuse

Offers one of the most up-to-date set of links to information and publications on substance abuse. Also a good source for statistics and publications.

World Wide Web:
   URL: **http://www.ccsa.ca/**

Change Assessment Research Project

For counselors and students, information on Prochaska and DiClementi's transtheoretical Model includes an excellent introduction to the model plus practical guides for its use. Also provides abstracts of current and past research projects, theses and dissertations and a master publications list.

World Wide Web:
   URL: **http://firenza.uh.edu/psychology/change/change.htm**

HabitSmart Medical

Offers links to information about addictive behavior, theories of habit endurance and habit change and tips for effectively managing problematic habitual behavior. Drug and alcohol abuse and adolescent experimentation is well covered. There are several self administered instruments, articles with suggestions for changing behaviour and a family page with information for parents and kids.

World Wide Web:
URL: **http://www.cts.com:80/~habtsmrt/**

Virtual Clearinghouse on Alcohol, Tobacco & Other Drugs

This site is a collaboration of a variety of organizations disseminating high quality information about the nature, extent and consequences of alcohol, tobacco and other drug use. It is available in English, French and Spanish. Includes a large selection of full-text documents, calendar of events and links to other sites.

World Wide Web:
URL: **http://www.ccsa.ca/atod/atod.htm**

Web of Addictions

Provides facts sheets on a variety of drugs in-depth information on specific topics, links to up-coming conferences, other resources and places to get help with addictions. This site is directed more at the public than health professionals, but still a good resource.

World Wide Web:
URL: **http://www.well.com/user/woa/**

Yahoo Drug List

Links to a variety of items including the Centre for Substance Abuse Prevention's "prevention Primer". It also links to Drugs Home Page which contains an immense amount of information about alcohol, drug tests and mind altering drugs(a bit offbeat).

World Wide Web:
URL: **http://www.yahoo.com/Entertainment/Drugs/**

Newsgroups

Usenet:
newsgroup: **alt.recovery**
newsgroup: **alt.abuse.recovery**

Listservers

DRUGABUS (related to drug abuse education information and research)
To join, send a message to **listserv@umab.umd.edu** with **sub drugabus** **<first name> <last name>** in the body of the message.

Addict-l
To join send mail to **listserv@kentvm.kent.edu** with **subscribe addict-l** **<first name> <last name>** in the body of message.

Aging

Administration on Aging: Internet and E-mail Resources on Aging

This is THE most extensive listing of resources related to aging, approximately 700! Sometimes referred to as the Post List.

World Wide Web:
URL: **http://www.aoa.dhhs.gov/aoa/pages/jpostlst.html**

GoldenAge Net

Offers links to resources related to long-term care and assisted living, commercial sites targeting seniors and their families, government sites, health sites and a directory of seniors' homepages.

World Wide Web:
URL: **http://elo.mediasrv.swt.edu/goldenage/intro.htm**

Health After 50

The Johns Hopkins Medical Letter is a monthly publication providing medical information and advice for those over 50. Selected articles from each issue are available at this site.

World Wide Web:
URL: **http://www.enews.com/magazines/jhml**

Institute on Aging at the University of Pennsylvania

In addition to links to other resources, this site offers the "Turtle Springs Virtual Seniors Community which provides health information, a newsstand, gazebo chat room and library. An interesting and colorful site!

World Wide Web:
  URL: **http://www.med.upenn.edu/%7Eaging/**

U.S. Administration on Aging: Directory of Web & Gopher Aging Sites

Links include governmental and non-governmental agencies, international sites, long-term care topics, mental health concerns, including Alzheimer's and related dementias, and libraries and databases.

World Wide Web:
  URL: **http://www.aoa.dhhs.gov/aoa/webres/craig.htm**

U.S. Seniors Resources

Offers links to non-profit organizations, guides and directories of interest to seniors in the U.S.

World Wide Web:
  URL: **http://www.contact.org/ussenior.htm**

Listservers

  GERINET
  To join   send mail to **listserv@UBMV.CC.BUFFALO.EDU** with **subscribe GERINET <first name> <last name>** in the body of message.

AIDS

AIDS and HIV Diseases

Links to other sites, many of the non-academic variety, announcements, directories, and organizations

World Wide Web:
    URL: **http://galaxy.einet.net/galaxy/Community/Health/Diseases/AIDS and HIV.html**

AIDS Resource List: Regional, National and International Sites

This site has many excellent links, however the choice of background color for the screens makes it difficult to look at for very long.

World Wide Web:
    URL: **http://www.teleport.com/%7Ecelinec/aids.shtml**

CDC National AIDS Clearinghouse

Includes current statistics, general information about prevention and treatment, workplace information and living with HIV, and surveillance reports.

World Wide Web:
    URL: **http://www.cdc.gov/cdc/html**

HIV: An Electronic Media Information Review

This site in Australia has excellent links to a wide variety of resources including fact sheets, international links, conference information and educational materials. Many of the information and links are also available in French, German, Italian and Spanish. It also has searching capabilities.

World Wide Web:
    URL: **http://florey.biosci.uq.edu.au/hiv/HIV_EMIR.html**

MedWeb: AIDS/HIV

This site only offers links to an extensive list of other resources. You could spend a lot of time browsing this site!

World Wide Web:
    URL: **http://www.gen.emory.edu/MEDWEB/keyword/ AIDS_and_HIV.html**

The National Institute of Allergy and Infectious Disease

Maintains a special section of its Gopher for AIDS information.

Gopher:
     Address: **odie.niaid.nih.gov.70/11/aids**
     Select: **Nursing HIV/AIDS**
     includes nursing practice, research, education, patient teaching and community care information

National Library of Medicine AIDS Information

Includes AIDSDRUGS database, Information Services for HIV/AIDS, and an extensive and current bibliography.

Gopher:
     URL: **gopher://gopher.nlm.nih.gov:70/11/aids**

WHO Global Programme on AIDS

Includes information related to this WHO initiative, epidemiology status and trends, women and AIDS, AIDS strategy, research and links to other sites

World Wide Web:
     URL: **http://gpawww.who.ch/gpahome.htm**
     Gopher:
     URL: **gopher://gpagopher.who.ch/**

WWW Virtual Library: AIDS

A virtual library page with links to sites dealing with the social, political, and medical aspects of AIDS. A good place to begin searching this topic. Some information on sexually transmitted diseases is also included

World Wide Web:
     URL: **http://golgi.harvard.edu/biopages/all.html**

Yahoo AIDS List

An excellent WWW site providing links to AIDS related information, resources centers, organizations, and an on-line version of the biweekly AIDS Information Newsletter.

World Wide Web:
URL: **http://www.yahoo.com/Health/Diseases_and_Conditions/**
AIDS_HIV

Newsgroups

Usenet:
newsgroup: **clari.tw.health.aids**
newsgroup: **misc.health.aids**
newsgroup: **sci.med.aids** (moderated)
newsgroup: HIV.AIDS.ARC
newsgroup: HIV.AIDS.LAW
newsgroup: HIV.AIDS.SPIRITUAL
newsgroup: HIV.AIDS.WOMEN
newsgroup: HIV.AIDS.DRUGS
newsgroup: HIV.AIDS.FR (French)
newsgroup: HIV.AIDS.SP (Spanish)

Allergies and Asthma

Allergy, Asthma & Immunology Online

This site is maintained by the American College of Allergy, Asthma & Immunology. It includes information for patients, physicians, news about allergy and
asthma, and links to other web sites. This site is searchable.

World Wide Web:
URL: **http://allergy.mcg.edu**

Allergy and Asthma Network/Mothers of Asthmatics, Inc.

Offers information on allergies and asthma, research news and information on
how to join this organization.

World Wide Web:
URL: **http://ww.podi.com/health/aanma**

Allergy and Asthma Web Page

This started as the **misc.kids** Allergy and Asthma FAQ so is geared toward the public, especially parents. Not an elegant site, but good information on re-sources, book reviews and an extensive collection of recipes

World Wide Web:
   URL: **http://cs.unc.edu/~kupstas/faq.html**

Allergy Clean Environments

Offers links to products and services for allergic individuals.

World Wide Web:
   URL: **http://www.w2.com:80/allergy.html**

The American Academy of Allergy, Asthma and Immunology

Provides general information, calendar of events. related organizations and agencies and scientific information resources.

World Wide Web:
   URL: **http://execpc.com/~edi/aaaai.html**

The Food Allergy Network

An excellent site for those with food allergies. Includes information, product alerts and updates, and a newsletter which includes allergy-free recipes and an-swers to diet dilemmas.

World Wide Web:
   URL: **http://www.foodallergy.org**

Latex Allergy Home Page

Includes advice from your allergist, a link to a management protocol and a link to a support organization.

World Wide Web:
   URL: **http://allergy.mcg.edu/physicians/ltxhome.html**

National Institute of Allergy and Infectious Diseases

Offers information about a wide variety of allergies and infectious diseases.

Gopher:
>URL: **gopher://gopher.niaid.nih.gov**

Newsgroups

Usenet:
>newsgroup: **alt.med.allergy**
>newsgroup: **alt.support.asthma**

Alternative Medicine

Health & Longevity: Naturopathy, Herbology, Nutrition, Homeopathy

Offers links to the current month's Newsletter, archives of past newsletters, and a health product catalogue.

World Wide Web:
>URL: **http://www.sims.net/organizations/naturopath/naturopath.html**

Homeopathy Home Page

Related to homeopathy and holistic medicine. It includes an FAQ explaining the difference between Western Medicine and homeopathy. Also included are a book list, e-mail address for two holistic listservs, and a homeopathic Internet Resource List.

World Wide Web:
>URL: **http://nearnet.gnn.com/wic/alt.01.html**
>URL: **http://www.dungeon.com/home/cam/homeo.html**

Homeopathic Internet Resource List

Links to networks, research, journals and organizations related to homeopathy.

World Wide Web:
    URL: **http://www.dungeon.com/home/cam/interlst.html**

Newsgroups:

Usenet:
    newsgroup: **misc.health.alternative**
    newsgroup: **alt.health.ayurveda**
    newsgroup: **soc.religion.shamanism**

Listservers

ALTMED-RES (Alternative medicine research)
    To join send mail to **majordomo@virginia.edu** with **subscribe ALTMED-RES <first name> <last name>** in the body of the message.

AROMA-TRIALS (Related to aromatherapy)
    To join send mail to **mailbase@mailbase.ac.uk** with **subscribe AROMA-TRIALS <first name> <last name>** in the body of the message.

Alzheimer's Disease

Alzheimer Web

Provides links to news items, research, articles, conferences and associations worldwide. General information can be accessed through the gopher site listed below.

World Wide Web:
    URL: **http://werple.mira.net.au/~dhs/ad.html**

Gopher:
    URL: **gopher://nisp.ncl.ac.uk:70/11/list-a-e/candid-dementia**

The Alzheimer Page

The Web page for the Alzheimer mailing list and its digest, Alzheimer-digest. Contains subscription information, searchable archives and links to related sites

World Wide Web:
   URL: **http://www.biostat.wustl.edu/alzheimer/**

Alzheimer's Disease Education & Referral Center

In addition to offering information, research and publications related to Alzheimer's Disease, there is also the ability to submit questions to be answered by specialists.

World Wide Web:
   URL: **http://www.cais.net/adear/**

Alzheimer's Disease Web Page

Contains links to resources for both family and professional caregivers. Also several links to neuropathology resources

World Wide Web:
   URL: **http://www.med.amsa.bu.edu/Alzheimer/home.html**

Listservers

ALZHEIMER
   To join, send mail to MARJORDOMO@WUBOIS.WUSTL.EDU with **subscribe ALZHEIMER <first name> <last name>** in the body of the message.

Arthritis

American College of Rheumatology Home Page

While largely offering services to its' members, this site also offers excellent patient information, an on-line version of "ACR News" and up-coming meetings

World Wide Web:
     URL: **http://www.rheumatology.org/**

Arthritis Foundation

A good place to start. Includes news and facts, a list of local offices, research resources and awards, information about "Arthritis Today", advocacy resources, information for health professional and a section on juvenile arthritis.

Anonymous FTP:
     Address: **ftp.netcom**
     Path: **/pub/arthritis/***

World Wide Web:
     URL: **ftp://ftp.netcom/pub/arthritis/arthritis.html**
     http://www.arthritis.org

HealthWeb: Rheumatology

Links to consumer and patient information, clinical trials, reference documents for health professional related to a variety of rheumatology topics including carpal tunnel syndrome, fibromyalgia and chronic fatigue syndrome.

World Wide Web:
     URL: **http://www.medlib.iupui.edu/cicnet/rheuma/disease.html**

Learning to Live with Arthritis

Management strategies for the person with arthritis. Practical information re-lated to a variety of topics such as diet, exercises, fatigue, pregnancy and travel.

World Wide Web:
     URL:
http://www.orthop.washington.edu/Bone%20and%20Joint%20Sources/xxx xxxxxz1_1.html (yes, 8 x's!)

National Institute of Arthritis and Musculoskeletal and Skin Diseases

Part of the National Institutes for Health, this site provides fact sheets, statistics, bibliographies, consensus conference reports, information on clinical trials, grants and news and events.

World Wide Web:
URL: **http://www.nih.gov/niams**

Newsgroups

Usenet:
newsgroup: **alt.support.arthritis**
newsgroup: **misc.health.arthritis**

Attention Deficit Disorder

Attention Deficit Disorder (ADD) Archive

Links to FAQ's, articles related to ADD, tips on living with ADD, mailing lists for parents and adults with ADD, and an ftp site where additional information and abstracts can be accessed.

World Wide Web:
URL: **http://www.seas.upenn.edu/~mengwong/add/**

Anonymous FTP:
Address: **ftp.mcs.com**
Path: **/mcsnet.users/falcon/add**

ADDNet

Full-text articles relating to interventions, particularly for educators.

Gopher:
 URL:**gopher://moe.coe.uga.edu:70/11/1TN%3A%Interactive% 20Teaching%20Network%20of%20UGA/A**

National Attention Deficit Disorder Association (ADDA)

This is a good starting point. Information related to parents, adults, legal concerns, employee assistance programs, medications, adult support groups, and an on-line journal for adults. Excellent links to other resources.

World Wide Web:
 URL: **http://www.add.org**
 Newsgroups
 Newsgroup: alt.support.attn-deficit

Breast Cancer

Breast Cancer Information Clearinghouse

Designed to provide information to patients and their families. Extensive links are provided to cancer listservs and other on-line information, medical information and support(organized by agency), subject oriented information (organized by topic), information for health professionals, support groups and upcoming conferences. The site to start with in searching for information about breast cancer.

World Wide Web:
 URL: **http://nysernet.org/bcic/**

National Breast Cancer Coalition Web Site

This is the Web site for a grassroots coalition formed to eradicate breast cancer through action and advocacy. Find information about current programs and new campaigns at this site.

World Wide Web:
 URL: **http://www.natbcc.org**

Oncolink

Provides information about the nature of cancer, breast self exam and mammography guidelines, psychological issues and risk factors.

World Wide Web:
    URL: **http://cancer.med.upenn.edu:80/1s/disease/breast**

Self Magazine's Breast Cancer Handbook

An on-line version of the magazine's breast cancer articles. It has a large multi-colored graphic on the home page that seems to take forever to load, so be patient.

World Wide Web:
    URL: **http://nysernet.org/bcic/self/**

Strang-Cornell Patient's Guide to Breast Cancer Treatment

Contains information about understanding breast cancer, mammography, making a diagnosis of breast cancer, surgical options, postoperative care, radiation therapy, reconstructive surgery, and family dynamics.

Gopher:
    Address: **nysernet.org**
    Port: **70**

World Wide Web:
    URL: **gopher://nysernet.org:70/11/BCIC/Sources/strang-cornell**

Cancer

CancerLit

Provides citations and abstracts on various cancer-related topics. Citations are added monthly.

Gopher:
    URL: **gopher://biomed.nus.sg:70/11/NUS-NCI-CancerNet/CLit**

CancerNet

World Wide Web:
>URL: **http://biomed.nus.sq/Cancer/welcome.html**
>A Web site that includes the following links

PDQ information statements on various types of cancer
>There are separate statements for physicians and patients. For patient teaching purposes, these information statements include a description of the type of cancer, staging, if appropriate and current treatment options for each stage. The location of other resources for patients is given. Physician and health care provider information includes clinical considerations, treatment options, treatments under clinical evaluation and references.

World Wide Web:
>URL: **http://biomed.nus.sg/Cancer/PhyPat.html**

PDQ supportive care statements
>which include suggested treatment protocols.

World Wide Web:
>URL: **http://biomed.nus.sg/Cancer/Supportive.html**

PDQ screening
>summaries provide current thinking on screening for various types of cancer. Extensive references are included.

World Wide Web:
>URL: **http://biomed.nus.sg/Cancer/Screening.html**

PDQ Drug Summaries
>highlight the pharmacologic composition , method of action, indications and extensive references.

World Wide Web:
>URL: **http://biomed.nus.sg/Cancer/Drugs.html**

CancerNet Cancer Articles

Contains four full text articles on self-managing cancer, specifically chemotherapy, home health management, relief from cancer pain and taking time

Gopher:
>URL: **gopher.nih.gov**
>Port: **70**

World Wide Web:
URL: **gopher://gopher.nih.gov:70/11/clin/cancernet/news/fulltext**

CancerNet News and General Information

World Wide Web:
URL: **http://biomed.sg/Cancer/General.html**

EINET Galaxy Cancer Page

Offers links to information about a variety of cancers for the medical professional.

World Wide Web:
URL: **http://galaxy.einet.net/galaxy/Medicine/**
Medical-Specialties/Cancer.html

Fact Sheets from the National Cancer Institute

Including Risk Factors, Prevention, Detection and Diagnosis, Cancer Site and Types, Cancer Therapy, Rehabilitation and Unconventional Methods

World Wide Web:
URL: **http://biomed.nus.sg/Cancer/Facts.html**

International Myeloma Foundation

Offers links to patient information, conferences, on-line articles, and a variety of other Internet resources related to cancer.

World Wide Web:
URL: **http://www.comed.com/IMF/imf.html**

OncoLink

Contains links to Disease Oriented menus, Specialty oriented menus, Psychological Support, Support Groups, Cancer Organizations, Spirituality, Clinical Trials, and other Cancer Resources.

World Wide Web:
   URL: **http://cancer.med.upenn.edu**

Talaria: The Hypermedia Assistant for Cancer Pain Management

Provides a hypermedia implementation of the Clinical Practice Guideline on the Management of Cancer Pain (U.S. Dept. of Health). Includes assessment guidelines, pharmacologic and non-pharmocologic management, non-pharmacologic interventions, a discussion of procedure-related pain in children and adults and a description of how to monitor the quality of pain management.

World Wide Web:
   URL: **http://www.stat.washington.edu/TALARIA/TALARIA.html**

Newsgroups

Usenet:
   newsgroup: **alt.support.cancer**
   newsgroup: **sci.med.diseases.cancer**

Listservers

CANCER-L (Public list for cancer-related issues)
   To join, send mail to **listserv@wvnvm.wvnet.edu** with **subscribe CANCER-L <first name> <last name>** in the body of the message.

Care Plans

Listservers

CAREPL-L (database of archived care plans
   To join, send a message to **CAREPL-L@UBVM.CC.BUFFALO.EDU** with **sub CAREPL-L <first name> <last name>** in the body of the message.

Celiac Disease

Celiac Discussion List Archives

As the title says, this archive contains on-line articles related to celiac disease, gluten-free diet information, links to the discussion list and to other resources.

World Wide Web:
    URL: **http://www.fastlane.net/homepages/thodge/archive.htm**

WWWebguides: Information for Gluten-free and Wheat-free Diets

Offers full text articles, recipes, support group information and commercial product information.

World Wide Web:
    URL: **http://www.wwwebguides.com/nutrition/diets/glutenfree**

Listservers

CELIAC
    To join, send a message to **listserv@sjuvm.st.johns.edu** with **sub CELIAC <first name> <last name>** in the body of the message.

Cel-Kids
    To join, send a message to **listserv@sjuvm.st.johns.edu** with CEL-KIDS **<first name> <last name>** in the body of the message.

Children's Health

Healthy Kids Magazine

Full-text articles from the current issue, plus archived issues.

World Wide Web:
    URL: **http://www.dc.enews.com/magazines/healthykids**

KidsHealth

Excellent information and resources for kids, parents and professionals related to a variety of topics including growth and development, nutrition, surgery, immunizations, lab tests and recipes.

World Wide Web:
　　URL: **http://KidsHealth.org**

Kids Nutrition

Good selection of full-text articles related to food safety, planning kids meals, feeding infants and making mealtimes pleasant.
　　gopher://tinman.mes.umn.edu:4242/11/ChildCare/Nutirion

Pediatric Points of Interest

Although it sounds medically-orientated, this site has good information for both the public and health care professionals. It includes links to an excellent and extensive number of organizations, articles and on-line "Ask a ...." consultations services related to parenting and specific diseases/conditions.

World Wide Web:
　　URL: **http://www.med.jhu.edu/peds/neonatology/poi.html**

Newsgroups

Usenet:
　　newsgroup: **misc.kids.health**

Listservers

PEDIATRIC-PAIN
　　To join, send mail to **mailserv@ac.dal.ca** with **subscribe PEDIATRIC-PAIN <first name> <last name>** in the body of the message.

Chronic Fatigue Syndrome

The Chronic Fatigue and Immune Dysfunction Syndrome Association of America

This is a well-maintained site offering information on CFIDS, Pediatric CFIDS, educational resources, an on-line newsletter and good links to other resources.

World Wide Web:
   URL: **http://www.ybi.com/cfids/index.html**

Chronic Fatigue Syndrome Electronic Newsletter

The current issue and back issues can be accessed through this page.

World Wide Web:
   URL: **http://www.alternatives.com/cfs-news/cfs-news.htm**

Chronic Fatigue Syndrome/Myalgic Encephalomyelitis

Provides information files, resources for health professional, listings of discussion groups and links to other resources.

World Wide Web:
   URL: **http://www.alternatives.com/cfs-news/index.htm**

The Facts About Chronic Fatigue Syndrome

This CDC site provides on-line information about possible causes, diagnosis, clinical aspects and demographics of CFS. CDC also maintains a 24 hour voice information system (404) 332-4555.

World Wide Web:
> URL: **http://www.cdc.gov/nicod/publications/cfs/cfshome.htm**

Newsgroups

Usenet:
> newsgroup: **alt.med.cfs**

Communicable Diseases

Centers for Disease Control

Provides extensive, searchable information and statistics related to prevention, incidence and immunization guidelines related to both common and unusual diseases. Includes guidelines for travelers.

World Wide Web:
> URL: **http://www.cdc.gov**

Communicable Diseases Fact Sheets

Provides information for the public on an extensive variety of communicable diseases

Gopher:
> URL: **gopher://gopher.health.state.ny.us/11/.consumer/.factsheets**

Health/Medical Internet Entry Points Directory: Communicable Diseases

Offers links to a wide variety of links to government sites, epidemiology information and public information.

World Wide Web:
> URL: **http://www.age.or.jp/x/akagi/healthep.htm**

Immunization Action Coalition

Offers information on immunization action.

World Wide Web:
URL: **http://www.immunize.org**

WWW Travel Health Information

Provides links to information about diseases, immunization environmental hazards, travel warnings and preventative measures.

World Wide Web:
URL: **http://www.intmed.mcw.edu/travel.html**

Community Health

Arizona Health Sciences Center Public Health Information Guide

Offers links to information about its course offerings and other related sites.

World Wide Web:
URL: **http://128.196.106.42/ph-hp.html**

Comprehensive Strategies for Health Promotion and Disease Prevention: Gateway to Related Internet Sites

Provides extensive links to health promotion strategies directed toward individuals, environmental change, and organizational development. Includes information related to workplace programs and community health promotion resources.
http://www.socecol.uci.edu/~socecol/depart/research/hpc/hpc-links.html

International Network for Interfaith Health Practices

Offers information, model practices and other health resources related to the interaction of faith and health. Particular resources for Parish Nurses

World Wide Web:
URL: **http://www.interaccess.com/ihpnet**

The "Virtual" Public Health Centre

Links to public health schools, courses and education resources, demography and population databases. Also extensive information related to a variety of public health topics. A good place to start searching this topic

World Wide Web:
    URL: **http://www-sci.lib.uci.edu/HSG/PHealth.html**

WHO Collaborating Center for Research on Healthy Cities

Links to current and archived newsletters, groups throughout the world and on-line information about the project.

World Wide Web:
    URL: **http://www.rulimburg.nl/~who-city/www.html**

Listservers

Community Mobilization/development
    To join, send an e-mail message to **listserv@zeus.med.uottawa.ca** with **subscribe community_mobilization/development <first name> <last name>** in the body of the message

General Community Health Issues
    To join, send an e-mail message to **listserv@zeus.med.uottawa.ca** with **subscribe general_community_health_issues <first name> <last name>** in the body of the message.

International Network for Interfaith Health Practices(formerly Parish Nurses)
    To join, send mail to **IHP-NET-REQUEST@synasoft**.com with **subscribe <first name> <last name>** in the body of the message.

PUBLIC-HEALTH
    To join, send mail to **mailbase@mailbase.ac.uk** with **subscribe PUBLIC-HEALTH <first name> <last name>** in the body of the message.

Rural-Care
> To join, send mail to **majordomo@avocado.pc.helsinki.fi with subscribe Rural-Care <first name> <last name>** in the body of the message.

RURALNET-L
> To join, send mail to **listserv@musom01.mu.wvnet.edu** with **subscribe RURALNET-L <first name> <last name>** in the body of the message.

Cystic Fibrosis

CF-WEB

Another site providing extensive information for both the public and health professionals, links to support groups, publications, up-coming conferences and the Archive of the Cystic-L mailing list.

World Wide Web:
> URL: **http://www.ai.mit.edu/people/mernst/cf/index.html**

Cystic Fibrosis Foundation

Provides information, news updates, clinical trial information, publications (some on-line) membership information and links to other resources.

World Wide Web:
> URL: **http://www.cff.org/index.html**

Cystic Fibrosis Resource Page

This page is intended to be an exhaustive guide to all web pages, mailing lists, FAQ's and newsgroups related to Cystic Fibrosis. It certainly lives up to its claims.

World Wide Web:
> URL: **http://vmsb.csd.mu.edu/~5418lukasr/cystic.html**

Listservers

Cystic-L
> To join, send mail to **listserv@Yalevm.cis.Yale.edu** with **subscribe cystic-l <first name> <last name>** in the body of the message.

Depression

Depression FAQ

Provides a FAQ (Frequently Asked Questions) list related to definitions and concepts, causes, treatment, medication, ECT, and relation to substance abuse and alcohol. The information could be used by the public or as an overview for health professionals.

World Wide Web:
   URL: **http://www.psych.helsinki.fi/~janne/asdfaq/index.html**

MentalHealth Net: Depression

This is the place to start looking for information related to depression. offers information for the public and health professionals, on-line articles, drug information, support group locations, assessment instruments and treatment guidelines.

World Wide Web:
   URL: **http://www.cmhc.com/guide/depress.htm**

Internet Depression Resources

Also offers good links to organizations, archives of several newsgroups and their respective FAQ's, direct links to subscribe to a variety of mailing lists, information on what to say and what not to say to a depressed person.

World Wide Web:
   URL: **http://stripe.colorado.edu/~judy/depression/**

Newsgroups

Usenet:
   newsgroup: **alt.psychology.help**
   newsgroup: **alt.support.depression**
   newsgroup: **alt.support.depression.manic**
   newsgroup: **alt.support.depression.seasonal**
   newsgroup: **alt.support.phobias**
   newsgroup: **sci.psychology**

newsgroup: **sci.med**
newsgroup: **sci.med.psycobiology**

Diabetes and Other Endocrine Disorders

Children with Diabetes

An on-line resource of kids and parents includes general information, a chat room, food and diet information, products and listings of other resources including camps.

World Wide Web:
URL: **http://www.castleweb.com/diabetes/index.html**

Diabetes Associations' Home pages

Provide information about the services offered by the various associations.

American Diabetes Association:

World Wide Web:
URL: **http://www.diabetes.org**

British Diabetic Association:

World Wide Web:
URL: **http://www.pavilion.co.uk/diabetic/**

Canadian Diabetes Association

World Wide Web:
URL: **http://www.diabetes.ca**

Juvenile Diabetes Foundation

World Wide Web:
URL: **http://www.jdfcure.com**

Diabetes on the Internet

Many links to associations, newsgroups, and other resources.

World Wide Web:
  URL: **http://www.minimed.com/files/dia_link.htm**

Diabetes Research International Network

Gopher:
  URL: **gopher://drinet.med.miami.edu:70/1**

NIH/NIDDK WEB Server

Provides links to diabetes statistics, control and complications trials, organizations, and information about diabetic eye disease, insulin dependent and non-insulin dependent diabetes.

World Wide Web:
  URL: **http://www.niddk.nih.gov/**

Patient Information Documents on Endocrine Disorders

Offers links to information about Addison's Disease, Cushing's Syndrome, and Familial Multiple Endocrine Neoplasia Type I.

World Wide Web:
  URL: **http://www.niddk.nih.gov/EndocrineDocs.html**

Newsgroups

Usenet:
  newsgroup: **misc.health.diabetes**
  newsgroup: **alt.support.diabetes.kids**

Listservers

DIABETES (International research project on diabetes)
  To join, send mail to **listserv@irlearn.ucd.ie** with **subscribe DIABETES <first name> <last name>** in the body of the message.

Digestive Diseases

Digestive Diseases Organizations

Directory of Digestive Diseases Organizations for Patients lists voluntary and private organizations involved in digestive diseases related activities, including provision of educational materials.

World Wide Web:
URL: **http://www.niddk.gov/DigDisOrgPat/DigDisOrgPat.html**

Directory of Digestive Diseases Organizations for Professionals lists organizations that represent health professionals involved in the study and treatment of digestive diseases.

World Wide Web:
URL: **http://www.niddk.nih.gov/DigDisOrgPro/DigDisOrgPro.html**

Patient Information Documents on Digestive Diseases

Offers links to patient education articles related to choosing a safe and successful weight loss program, constipation, heartburn, hemorrhoids, and lactose intolerance.

World Wide Web:
URL: **http://www.niddk.nih.gov:80/DigestiveDocs.html**

Newsgroups

Usenet:
newsgroup: **alt.support.crohns-colitis**

Disabilities

ABLEDATA: The National Database of Assistive Technology Information

An extensive database listing information on assistive technology available both commercially and non-commercially. It offers fact sheets and its own "top ten" searches.

Gopher:
> URL: **gopher.//val-dor.cc.buffalo.edu:70/11/.naric/.abledata**

Aztech

Includes links to Assistive Technology resources for consumers, Technical and general market resources, Supporting Organizations, both governmental and non-profit and information and referral.

Gopher:
> URL: **gopher://cosmos.ot.buffalo.edu:80/hGET%20/aztech.html**

CODI: Cornucopia of Disability Information

A well maintained repository for disability related information of all types

Gopher:
> URL: **gopher://val-dor.cc.buffalo.edu**

Communication Disorders & Sciences

Outlines the Internet resources available on communication disorders

Gopher:
> URL: **gopher://una.hh.lib.umich.edu:70/00/inetdirsstacks/ commdis%3Akuster**

CooL Disability Resources on the Internet

Links to a variety of other Web sites, general, educational and government re-sources. This is a good place to begin a search related to disabilities.

World Wide Web:
  URL: **http://disability.com/cool.html**

Deaf Gopher

Actually a WWW site. Contains information about deaf education resources, electronic resources and general deafness information, including development of deaf children. A gopher site to access if you don't have Web facilities is noted below.

World Wide Web:
  URL: **http://web.cal.msu.edu/deaf/deafintro.html**

Gopher:
  URL: **gopher://burrow.cl.msu.edu:70/11/msu/dept/deaf**

Deaf WWW server

Offers information about educational resources, electronic deaf resources, and general deaf information. It includes special education class descriptions and syllabi from Michigan State University.

World Wide Web:
  URL: **http://web.cal.msu.edu/deaf/deafintro.html**

DISABILITY Resources on the Internet

Another good place to search for information related to disabilities. This WWW site has links to a variety of organizations, newsletters, and articles related to a variety of disabilities.

World Wide Web:
  URL: **http://www.eskimo.com/~jlubin/disabled.html**

Dyslexia

An excellent place to start looking for resources related to dyslexia. This page has numerous links to other sites, information related to education, support and other organizations and associations.

World Wide Web:
  URL: **http://www.iscm.ulst.ac.uk/~george/subjects/dyslexia.html**

Yahoo Disabilities List

Extensive links to Web sites related to a variety of disabilities. The links include newsletters, organizations, and institutes. Many of these resources are more oriented to health professionals.

World Wide Web:
URL: **http://www.yahoo.com**
Society_and_Culture/Disabilities/

Newsgroups

Usenet:
newsgroup: **misc.handicap**
newsgroup: **alt.support.dev-delays**
newsgroup: **alt.support.cerebral-palsy**
newsgroup: **alt.support.spina-bifida**

Listservers

bit.listserv.autism
Children with special health care needs To join, send mail to **listserv@nervm.nerdc.ufl.edu** with **subscribe cshcn <first name> <last name>** in the body of the message.

Down Syndrome

Down Syndrome

An excellent starting point. Links to organizations and associations, Archives of the Down Syndrome Listserv, on-line articles, and medical resources.

World Wide Web:
URL: **http://www.oise.on.ca/~bglenn/down.html**

Down Syndrome WWW Page

Offers links to contributed articles, a medical checklist, worldwide organizations, inclusion and educational resources, parent matching and support groups, conferences, and toy catalogues

World Wide Web:
　　URL: **http://www.nas.com/downsyn/**

Parents Helping Parents

Links to LINCS, a searchable on-line human services directory addressing the needs of children and adults with most any need for specialized care or services. For those without WWW access, there is an FTP site.

World Wide Web:
　　URL: **http://www.php.com**

Anonymous FTP:
　　Address: **ftp.netcom.com**
　　Login: **anonymous**
　　Password: **your e-mail address**
　　Path: **/pub/LI/LINCS**

Listservers

bit.listserv.down-syn
　　Children with Down Syndrome. To join, send mail to **listserv@vm1. nodak.edu** with **subscribe down-syn <first name> <last name>** in the body of the message

Eating Disorders

Anorexia: Information for Patients, Family & Friends

Although this site is aimed at the public, there is good information for health professionals also. There are links to a wide variety of resources and support groups, information about recognition and treatment.

World Wide Web:
　　URL: **http://www.neca.com/~cwildes/**

Eating Disorders

Aimed at the general public. It includes information about eating disorders, symptoms, a self-assessment questionnaire, and tips for resolution.

World Wide Web:
    URL: **http://ccwf.cc.utexas.edu/~bjackson/UTHealth/eating.html**

Internet Mental Health: Anorexia Nervosa: Research Re: Treatment

Full-text articles about current research related to treatment of eating disorders.

World Wide Web:
    URL: **http://www.mentalhealth.com/dis-rs2/p25-et01.html**

Newsgroups

Usenet:
    newsgroup: **alt.support.eating-disord**

Emergency Medical Services (EMS)

Emergency Medical Services Home Page

Provides links to other Internet sites of interest to EMS including pharmacology, emergency medicine and a health information newsletter.

World Wide Web:
    URL: **http://galaxy.tradewave.com/galaxy/Community/
    Health/Emergency-Medicine/fritz-nordengren/ems.html**

Emergency Nursing World

A large site with links of interest to all EMS practitioners. Includes tips and tricks, pediatric hints discharge instructions, links to other sites, mailing lists and newsgroups

World Wide Web:
    URL: **http://www.hooked.net/~ttrimble/enw/enw_toc.html**

Listservers

EMED-L

Hospital-based emergency medical practitioners. To join send mail to **list-serv@itssrv1.ucsf.edu** with **sub EMED-L <first name> <last name>** in the body of the message

INJURY-L

To join send mail to **listserv@wvnvm.wvnet.edu** with **sub injury-l <first name> <last name>** in the body of the message

Newsgroups

Usenet:

newsgroup: **misc.emergency.services**
newsgroup: **misc.ems**

Endometriosis

Mental Health Net: Self-Help Resources: Endometriosis

Offers on-line information about causes, symptoms, diagnosis and treatment and addresses for associations.

World Wide Web:
URL: **http://www.cmhc.com/factsfam/endo.htm**

Listservers

WITSENDO

To join send mail to **listserv@dartcms1.dartmouth.edu** with **sub WITSENDO <first name> <last name>** in the body of the message.

Epilepsy

Epilepsy Link Page

Offers extensive links to other resources, support groups and organizations, information, medications, discussion groups and mailing lists.

World Wide Web:
URL: **http://www.gatecom.com/~jlyon/epil.html**

The Epilepsy Link Page

Offers information, current news, links to other resources, including discussion groups and mailing lists.

World Wide Web:
URL: **http://www.neuro.wustl.edu/epilepsy/links.html**

Listservers

Epilepsy-List (for persons living with Epilepsy and their families)
To join, send mail to **listserv@calvin.dgbt.doc.ca** with **subscribe epilepsy-list <first name> <last name>** in the body of the message.

Epilepsy-Pro (for professionals)
To join, send mail to **listserv@calvin.dgbt.doc.ca** with **subscribe epilepsy-pro <first name> <last name>** in the body of the message.

Newsgroups

Usenet:
newsgroup: **alt.support.epilepsy**

Ethics

Centerviews

Is the newsletter of the Center for Biomedical Ethics, School of Medicine, Case Western Reserve University. Includes full-text articles, archived articles, and a calendar of upcoming events.

World Wide Web:
   URL: **http://www.cwu.edu/CWRU/Dept/Med/bioethics/centerviews.html**

Listservers

BIOMED-L (Related to biomedical ethics)
   To join, send mail to **listserv@VM1.NODAK.Edu** with **subscribe BIOMED-L <first name> <last name>** in the body of the message.

Evidence Based Practice

Center for Evidence-based Medicine

Includes a "toolbox", teaching archives, information about the Center and its publications.

World Wide Web:
   URL: **http://cebm.jr2.ox.ac.uk**

The Clinical Evaluation Research Group

Focused on evaluation of advanced practice within specialist roles, psychological and educational interventions by nurses and wound care and infection control. Topics are identified with the group member and links are available to the researcher.

World Wide Web:
   URL:
   http://www.kcl.ac.uk/kis/schools/life_sciences/nursing/CEVAL.html

Cochrane Collaboration on Effective Professional Practice

Offers a newsletter and checklist that can be downloaded. Seems to be still under development, but a site to watch.

World Wide Web:
URL: **http://www.york.ac.uk/inst/ccepp/welcome.htm**

EvidenceBased Health

A good place to begin browsing this topic. Includes links to international sites related to evidence-based practice.

World Wide Web:
URL: **http://www.ki.se/phs/hprin/hprin7.htm**

Fibromyalgia

Fibromyalgia Resources

Good links to other resources including related health information, research and associations

World Wide Web:
URL: **http://www.azstarnet.com/~mccrull/fibro.html**

National Fibromyalgia Research Association

Offers links to diagnostic criteria, exercise guidelines and information resources.

World Wide Web:
URL: **http://www.telport.com/~nfra**

A Physician's Guide to Fibromyalgia Syndrome

Although directed at physicians, there is good information for other health care professionals, including etiology, diagnosis, treatment and a table of useful drugs.

World Wide Web:
   URL: **http://www.hsc.missouri.edu/fibro/fm-md.html**

Newsgroups

Usenet:
   newsgroup: **alt.med.fibromyalgia**

Listservers

FIROM-L
   To join, send a message to **listserv@vmd.cso.uiuc.edu** with **sub FIROM-L <first name> <last name>** in the body of the message.

Gerontology

Aging Research Center

Provides links to full-text articles related to various theories of aging, up-coming conferences, newsgroups and journals.

World Wide Web:
   URL: **http://www.hookup.net:80/mall/aging/agesit59.html**

MedWeb: Geriatrics

Extensive links to resources covering all aspects of geriatrics, such as cardiology, dentistry, mental health, osteoporosis and stroke.

World Wide Web:
   URL: **http://www.gen.emory.edu/MEDWEB/keyword/Geriatrics.html**

Listservers

Fall prevention in the elderly
   To join, send an e-mail message to **listserv@zeus.med.uottawa.ca** with **subscribe fall_prevention_in_the_elderly <first name> <last name>** in the body of the message.

GERINET

>To join, send a message to **listserv@ubvm.cc.buffalo.edu-bit.listserv. GERINET** with **subscribe GERINET <first name> <last name>** in the body of the message.

Grief

Death, Dying and Grief Resources

This is an extensive index of Internet resources related to bereavement and grief including newsgroups, children and family support, and healing.

World Wide Web:
>URL: **http://www.cyberspy.com/~webster/death.htm#general**

GriefNet

Provides good links to resources for both bereaved persons and healthcare professionals, an excellent collection of on-line articles including sections related to children, families and pets, and an extensive list of on-line support groups.

World Wide Web:
>URL: **http://rivendell.org/**

Listservers

grief-chat

>To join, send mail to **majordomo@falcon**.ic.net with **subscribe grief-chat <first name> <last name>** in the body of the message.(There are many specialized groups at this site. This list will help you to connect to a suitable group)

Newsgroups

Usenet:
>newsgroup: **alt.support.grief**
>newsgroup: **soc.support.pregnancy.loss**

Headache

Excedrin Headache Resource Center

Offers advice on tracking and evaluating headaches, management and lifestyle headache triggers. Includes a Headache Workbook and Headache Diary.

World Wide Web:
URL: **http://womenslink.com/wlink/health/quality/excedrin.html**

Headache Archive

Archives of the mailing list dating from 1994. Provides information about the physical, emotional, social and economic impact of headaches.

Anonymous FTP:
Address: **niord.shsu.edu**
Path: **/headache.dir/***

Migraine Resource Center

Offers articles related to triggers, symptoms, treatment programs, diagnostic screening and latest news.

World Wide Web:
URL: **http://www.migrainehelp.com**

Listservers

headache
To join, send mail to **listserv@shsu.edu** with **subscribe headache <first name> <last name>** in the body of the message.

Newsgroups

Usenet:
newsgroup: **alt.support.headaches.migraine**

Health

Canadian Society for International Health

Links to other organizations and an FTP site for accessing CSIH documents.

World Wide Web:
 URL: **http://www.hwc.ca**

Hardin Meta Directory of Internet Health Sources

This directory contains extensive links to sites directed at both the public and health care professionals related to a variety of topics noted by medical specialty.

World Wide Web:
 URL: **http://ww3.arcade.uiowa.edu/hardin-www/md.html**

Healthline

Offers information for the lay person on a variety of health topics including exercise, diet drug and alcohol abuse and sexuality.

World Wide Web:
 URL: **http://www.healthline.umt.edu.700**

HealthNet

Has the goal of providing one window of access to all health-related Internet resources. There are extensive links to other sites. An excellent place to start browsing.

World Wide Web:
 URL: **http://debra.dgbt.doc.ca/`mike/home.html**

Health-related World Wide Web Server

Offers links to an extensive variety of other WWW sites related to health. A favorite spot to begin browsing!

World Wide Web:
URL: **http://www.who.ch/others/OtherHealthWeb.html**

Health Resources

Provides links to numerous heath-related Web sites. This is a good place to check for newly developed sites. One of our favorites!

World Wide Web:
URL: **http://gnn.com/wic/wics/med.new.htmll**

HealthWeb

Provides "organized access to evaluated, non-commercial" Internet resources. A key to this site is that the resources included are evaluated, so standards have been applied to the offerings. There is an extensive listing of topics.

World Wide Web:
URL: **http://www.ghsl.nwu.edu/healthweb/**

Healthwise (a program of Columbia University)

Has links to "Dear Alice" questions and answers related to sexual health and relationships, drug and alcohol concerns, nutrition, emotional well-being and general health. Users can submit questions on-line. This is easily read information for the public.

World Wide Web:
URL: **http://www.columbia.edu/cu/healthwise/**

Internet Health Newsgroups and Listserver Groups

Provides links to a large variety of newsgroups and listserver groups arranged by health topic. This is a good place to check for new groups that are not found in this catalogue.

World Wide Web:
URL: **http://www.ihr.com/newsgrp.html**

Magellan: Health and Medicine

Extensive links to a large variety of health resources such as conditions and diseases, personal fitness, personal care, services and resources. Another excellent place to start browsing. This is a searchable site.

World Wide Web:
  URL: **http://www.mckinley.com/browse_bd.cgi?health**

National Institutes of Health

Offers information on a variety of health topics and also clinical information.

World Wide Web:
  URL: **http://www.nih.gov**

Yahoo: Health

Probably the best place to start looking for health-related information. Examples of links include diseases and conditions, education, fitness, general health, health administration, mental health reproductive health sexuality and workplace health. This site is searchable.

World Wide Web:
  URL: **http://www.yahoo.com/health/**

Newsgroups

Usenet:
  newsgroup: **clari.tw.health**

Listservers

HEALTH-L (related to health research)
  To join, send mail to **listserv@irlearn.ucd.ie** with **subscribe HEALTH-L
  <first name> <last name>** in the body of the message.

HealthNet Listserv
  To join, send mail to **listserv@calvin.dgbt.doc.ca** with **subscribe healthnet <first name><last name>** in the body of the message.

Health Promotion

Good Medicine Magazine

Provides on-line access to the current edition of this publication which focuses on preventative medicine combining both traditional and holistic practices.

World Wide Web:
URL: **http://none.coolware.com/health/good_med/ThisIssue.html**

Health Promotion

Provides sub-menus that provide information at a lay level to assist individuals to plan and carry out health promotion activities. Sub-menus relate to back and neck care, body image, breast self-exam, eye care, fast food calorie counter, health promotion suggested timetable, massage, relationships, and testicular self-exam.

World Wide Web:
URL: **http://www.uiuc.edu/departments/mckinley/health-info/hlthpro/hlthpro.html**

Listservers

Behaviour Change Strategies
To join, send an e-mail message to **listserv@zeus.med.uottawa.ca** with **subscribe behavioural_change_strategies <first name> <last name>** in the body of the message.

FIT-L
To join, send a message to **listserv@etsuadm.etsu.edu** with **sub fit-l <first name> <last name>** in the body of the message.

Newsgroups

Usenet:
newsgroup: **misc.fitness**
newsgroup: **su.org.hpp-aerobics**

Heart Health

American Heart Association

Offers on-line articles including "Heart & Stroke A to Z Guide, risk assessment, lists of local resources and information for health professionals.

World Wide Web:
URL: **http://www.amhrt.org/index.html**

Arnot Ogden Medical Center: Heart Health

This is an excellent resource for patient teaching materials. There are extensive on-line articles written for the lay person related to all aspects of cardiovascular disease, prevention, surgery and rehabilitation. Searchable.

World Wide Web:
URL: **http://www.aomc.org/HOD2/general/heart-Contents.html**

Home Health

Eldercare Web

Includes information on home health and day care services, articles related to decision-making about housing options, assisted living alternatives and information for families.

World Wide Web:
URL: **http://www.ice.net/~kstevens/living.htm**

The Home Care Web Page

Grew out of the hcarenurs listserv. Contains information targeted to home care and hospice nurses, including links to other sites.

World Wide Web:
URL: **http://junior.apk.net/~nurse/**

National Association for Home Care

Offers consumer information, lists of associations, vendor lists, an on-line version of "Caring" magazine, including archives and a listing of up-coming meetings.

World Wide Web:
 URL: **http://www.nahc.org**

Listservers

hcarenurse
 To join send e-mail to **majordomo@po.cwru.edu** with **subscribe hcarenurse <your e-mail address>** in the body of the message.

homehlth
 To join send e-mail to **listserv@usa.net** with **subscribe homehlth <first-name> <last-name>** in the body of the message.

HOSPICE
 To join send e-mail to **majordomo@po.cwru.edu** with **subscribe hospice <your e-mail address>** in the body of the message.

Hospitals

Hospitals on the World Wide Web

Has links to a variety of hospitals around the world. The information provided by the various hospitals is not consistent, but may include department information, site plans and telephone listings.

World Wide Web:
 URL: **http://neuro-www.mgh.harvard.edu/hospitalweb.nclk**

Yahoo: Health: Hospitals

Also provides links to hospitals, subdivided into children's hospitals, colleges and universities, military and Veterans Affairs Hospitals.

World Wide Web:
 URL: **http://www.yahoo.com/Health/Hospitals/**

Immune System Disorders

Ask an Immunologist

The introduction to this site says that anyone from high school students to university professors can ask related questions. This is not a resource for solving personal health problems, rather general information related to immune system disorders or immunology.

World Wide Web:
   URL: **http://glamdring.ucsd.edu/other/aai/askAAI.html**

Lupus Foundation of America

Offers a detailed FAQ, current information, research library, lists of support groups and agencies and information related to causes, symptoms, testing and treatment.

World Wide Web:
   URL: **http://www.lupus.org/lupus/**

Listservers

IMMUNE
   To join, send e-mail message **to IMMUNE-REQUEST@WEBER. UCSD.EDU** with **subscribe IMMUNE <first name> <last name>** in the body of the message.

Informatics

AMIA: Nursing Informatics Working Group

Provides information on current activities, education in nursing informatics, upcoming conferences and links to related sites

World Wide Web:
   URL: **http://www.gl.umbc.edu/~abbott/nurseinfo.html**

COACH: Canada's Health Informatics Association

General information, publications and conference announcements are found here. Also links to other resources.

World Wide Web:
URL: **http://www.agt.net/public/coachorg/**

Duke Medical Informatics

Provides links to other health and medical informatics links worldwide.

World Wide Web:
URL: **http://dmi-www.mc.duke.edu/**

St. F.X.U. Nursing Informatics

This site offers extensive links to health care informatics sites worldwide. Definitely the place to start searching this topic. Also excellent links to general nursing and health care sites.

World Wide Web:
URL: **http://juliet.stfx.ca/people/fac/mackinn/nursei.html**

The Webster: Nursing Informatics

Another large list of on-line resources, including national and international organizations.

World Wide Web:
URL: **http://ally.ios.com/~webster/nurse.html#informatics**

Newsgroups

Usenet:
newsgroup: **sci.med.informatics**

Listservers

CPRI-L (related to telecommunications in healthcare)
To join, send a message to **listserv@ukanaix.cc.ukans.edu** with **subscribe CPRI-L <first name> <last name>** in the body of the message.

MEDINF-L
To join send mail to **listserv@vm.gmd.de** with **subscribe MEDINFO-L <first name> <last name>** in the body of the message.

Nursing Informatics
To join, send a message to **listproc@lists.umass.edu** with **subscribe nrsing-l <first name> <last name>** in the body of the message.

Job Search

MedSearch America

Provided by a commercial service; allows you to post your resume on-line, search jobs and search resumes. Also includes information about health care industry resources, career articles and outlook.

World Wide Web:
URL: **http://www.medsearch.com**

Kidney & Urologic Disorders

Directory of Kidney and Urologic Diseases Organizations

Provides a list of voluntary, governmental and private organizations(including addresses and telephone numbers) involved in kidney and urologic disease related activity.

World Wide Web:
URL: **http:/www.niddk.nih.gov/**
KidneyOrganizations/KidneyOrganizations.html

The International Society for Peritoneal Dialysis

Information is available in English, French, Italian and Spanish. Includes meeting/conference announcements, recommendations for training, for treatment of peritonitis, a page for nurses, nutritionists and social workers and a patient's page.

World Wide Web:
   URL: **http://www.ispd.org/**

Kidney and Urologic Diseases Database

This is a searchable database of health promotion and educational materials related to this topic.

World Wide Web:
   URL: **http://www.aerie.com/nihdb/nkudic/kudbase.html**

National Institute of Diabetes, Digestive and Kidney Disease

Information about various diseases for the public, research information, facts and statistics for health care professionals.

World Wide Web:
   URL: **http://www.niddk.nih.gov/NIDDK_HomePage.html**

Patient Education Documents on Kidney Diseases

Provides links to information about end-stage renal disease and treatment choices, kidney diseases, kidney stones, and polycystic kidneys. Also links to professional and voluntary organizations and the U.S. Renal Data System statistics.

World Wide Web:
   URL: **http://www.niddk.nih.gov/KidneyDocs.html**

Patient Education Documents on Urological Diseases

Offers information related to impotence, interstitial cystitis, prostate enlargement and urinary tract infection. Also professional and voluntary organizations.

World Wide Web:
  URL: **http://www.niddk.nih.gov/UrologicDocs.html**

Medical Technology

The Medical Technology Page

Provides medical technology briefs on topics such as 3_d Visualization of Fetal Ultrasound, Mammography, and Near-field Optical Microscopy

World Wide Web:
  URL: **http://w3.pnl.gov:2080/medical/**

Listservers

MED-TECH
  To join send mail to **listerv@vm1.ferris.edu** with **subscribe MED-TECH <first name> <last name>** in the body of the message.

Menopause

A Friend Indeed

Provides menopause information and articles and subscription information for the newsletter "A Friend Indeed".

World Wide Web:
  URL: **http://www.odyssee.net/~janine**

MedAccess: Menopause

Provides on-line articles related to effects of menopause, managing menopause, on-going research and organizations and resources.

World Wide Web:
  URL: **http://www.medaccess.com/physical/menop/meno_toc.htm**

Menopause

This is an excellent site to begin searching this topic. Information related to Estrogen Replacement Therapy, NIH menopause articles, monitoring bone loss, and osteoporosis.

World Wide Web:
URL: **http://www.ivf.com/meno.html**

Newsgroups

Usenet:
newsgroup: **alt.support.menopause**

Mental Health

Florida Mental Health Institute

Links to its research and demonstration projects in the areas of Aging and mental health, Child and family studies, Community mental health and Mental health law and policy.

World Wide Web:
URL: **http://www.fmhi.usf.edu/**

Mental Health Net: Professional Resources

Information related to associations and organizations, DSM criteria, journals, mailing lists and newsgroups with specific interests. Searchable by topic.

World Wide Web:
URL: **http://www.cmhc.com/prof.htm**

Mood Disorders

Has extensive links to information and other sites related to depression, seasonal affective disorder(SAD), medication and transmitters and a depression FAQ.

World Wide Web:
URL: **http://www.psych.helsinki.fi/~janne/mood/mood.html**

National Institutes of Mental Health

Information related to grants and contracts, publications, on-line education programs, and consensus conference proceedings. For both the public and health care professionals.

World Wide Web:
   URL: **http://www.nimh.nih.gov**

Gopher:
   URL: **gopher://gopher.nimh.nih.gov:70**

Obsessive-Compulsive Disorder

Has links to medical resources, personal resources, other on-line services, definitions and a bulletin board.

World Wide Web:
   URL: **http://mtech.csd.uwm.edu/~fairlite/ocd.html**

PsychNET: American Psychological Association

Maintained by the American Psychological Association, this site offers information for the public, public policy/advocacy information, selected articles from the APA Monitor, science, education and practice information. Also includes information about up-coming conferences and information for APA members. Searchable.

World Wide Web:
   URL: **http://www.apa.org**

Seasonal Affective Disorder

Provides a list of print resources about SAD, organizations and information about light sources..

World Wide Web:
   URL: **http://www.psych.helsinki.fi/~janne/mood/sad.html**
A technical FAQ on Seasonal Affective Disorder is available through

Anonymous FTP:
   Address: **ftp.std.com**
   Path: **/pub/walkers**

Yahoo Internet Mental Health Resources

Provides links to information on a variety or medical and mental health topics.

World Wide Web:
   URL: **http://www.yahoo.com/Health/Mental_Health/**

Listservers

PSYCHOPHYSIOLOGY
   To join, send a message to **MAILBASE@MAILBASE.AC.UK** with
   JOIN CLINICAL-PSYCHOPHYSIOLOGY in the body of the message.

Newsgroups

Usenet:
   newsgroup: **sci.med.psychobiology**
   newsgroup: **sci.psychology**
   newsgroup: **alt.society.mental-health**
   newsgroup: **alt.psychology.personality**
   newsgroup: **alt.sexual.abuse.recovery**
   newsgroup: **alt.support.dissociation**

Mental Retardation

The Arc Home Page

Offers links to The Arc's government reports, publications, fact sheets and listings of other Internet resources. Also included is specific information related to
ageing and mental retardation and fetal alcohol syndrome.

World Wide Web:
   URL: **http://fohnix.metronet.com/~thearc/welcome.html**

Resources on Mental Retardation

On-line articles, information about organizations, and special Olympics. Good
links to other resources and information including a list of mailing lists for a
variety of concerns related to this topic.

World Wide Web:
   URL:
   http://curry.edschool.virginia.edu/curry/dept/cise/ose/categories/mr.html

SERI: Special Education Resources on the Internet

Collections of Internet accessible information and resources largely focused on education.

World Wide Web:
   URL: **http://www.hood.edu/seri/**

Midwifery, Pregnancy and Childbirth

The Breastfeeding Page

On-line articles and information in both English and Spanish, including initiating feeding, sore nipple management, and extensive links to other resources. A good place to start!

World Wide Web:
   URL: **http://www.islandnet.com/~bedford/brstfeed.html**

Midwifery, Pregnancy and Birth Related Information

Provides links to information about the history of midwifery, homebirths, nutrition and pregnancy, lactation, breastfeeding and infant nutrition. There are also links to Midwifery Today's list of e-mail addresses. This is THE place to start looking for information on this topic

World Wide Web:
   URL: **http://www.efn.org/~djz/birth/birthindex.html**

Midwifery Today

Articles are available on-line.

World Wide Web:
   URL: http://**nightingale.con.utk.edu:70/11/**
   Publications/Periodicals/midwif-articles

MIDWIFE WWW Home Page

Has links to a variety of types of information related to midwifery including doulas, birth methods, breastfeeding, e-mail lists, and conferences.

World Wide Web:
   URL: **http://med714.bham.ac.uk/nursing/midwife/**

Gopher:
   URL: **gopher -p/papers/nurse.csv.warwick.ac.uk**

World Wide Web:

Listservers

MIDWIFE
   To join, send mail to **midwife-request@fensende.com** with **subscribe MIDWIFE <first name> <last name>** in the body of the message.

FET-NET (Research in fetal and perinatal care)
   To join, send mail to **LISTSERV@HEARN.BITNET** with **SUB FET-NET <first name> <last name>** in the body of the message.

PRENAT-L
   To join, send mail to **LISTSERV@ALBNYDH2.BITNET** with **SUB PRENAT-L <first name> <last name>** in the body of the message.

Newsgroups

Usenet:
   newsgroup: **misc.kids.health**
   newsgroup: **misc.kids.pregnancy**
   newsgroup: **misc.kids.breastfeeding**
   newsgroup: **alt.support.breastfeeding**
   newsgroup: **alt.infertility**

Multiple Sclerosis

Autoimmunity Research

This is a good research information source, however, the contrast and print is of very poor quality, making it a challenge to get to the useful information.

World Wide Web:
    URL: **http://www.cps.msu.edu/keyesdav/ms/**

Multiple Sclerosis Society of Canada

Offers links to information about MS, a discussion area and latest research.

World Wide Web:
    URL: **http://www.ncf.carleton.ca/freeport/social.services/ms/menu**

National Multiple Sclerosis Society

A good selection of on-line information about MS, plus links to other organizations and resources.

World Wide Web:
    URL: **http://www.nmss.org**

Newsgroups

Usenet:
    newsgroup: **alt.support.mult-sclerosis**

Neuroscience

Neurosciences on the Internet

This is THE site to browse a variety of topics such as brain injury and spinal cord injury.

World Wide Web:
    URL: **http://www.lm.com/~nab**

Nutrition

Arizona Health Sciences Library Nutrition Guide

Includes links to foods and nutrition information, food technology, food labeling, nutrient data, clip art, newsletters and educational resources. This is a very large index.

World Wide Web:
URL: **http://www.medlib.arizona.edu/educ/nutrition.html**

Centre for Food Safety and Nutrition

Provides links to information related to biotechnology, consumer advice, foodborne illness, food labeling, and FDA regulations.

World Wide Web:
URL: **http://vm.cfsan.fda.gov/list.html**

CSIRO Division of Human Nutrition

Offers links to an extensive variety of other resources and sites including consumer leaflets and research. A good site to browse.

World Wide Web:
URL: **http://www.dhn.csiro.au**

ElNet Galaxy Nutrition Index

Provides links to searches of nutrition-related topics and educational programs.

World Wide Web:
URL: **http://galaxy.einet.net/Medicine/Health-Occupations/
Nutrition.html**

Food and Nutrition Information Center

Extensive links to publications, databases, full-text articles, FDA/USDA guidelines and other Internet resources.

World Wide Web:
URL: **http://www.nal.usda.gov/fnic**

Godiva On-line

This is a Web site of Godiva chocolates. This is a fun (if not nutritious) site to visit. It offers links to the history of chocolate as well as recipes and on-line ordering!

World Wide Web:
URL: **http://www.godiva.com**

Index of Food and Nutrition Internet Resources

This is a huge list of links to on-line food and nutrition information related to specific diseases and conditions. It also includes research, statistics and software links

World Wide Web:
URL: **http://www.nalusda.gov/fnic/fnic-extexts.html**

International Food Information Council

A Web site with the bulk of the links organized according to audience (parents, educators, etc.) related to subjects such as caffeine, food coloring, biotechnology, pregnancy, hyperactivity and aspartame. Especially good consumer education.

World Wide Web:
URL: **http://ificinfo.health.org/**

Purdue Food Science Home Page

Offers links to the Computer Integrated Food Manufacturing Center, the Whistler Center for Carbohydrate Research, conferences, courses and other food science-related resources.

World Wide Web:
URL: **http://www.foodsci.purdue.edu/Text/index.htm**

The No Milk Page

This is a good staring point for information related to lactose intolerance, milk allergy or casein intolerance.

World Wide Web:
   URL: **http://www.panix.com/~nomilk/**

Vegetarian Recipes

Contains a searchable index and list of over 1200 vegetarian recipes.

World Wide Web:
   URL: **http://www-sc.ucssc.indiana.edu/cgi-bin/recipes/**

Yahoo Nutrition Page

Offers links to a variety of nutrition sites and information.

World Wide Web:
   URL: **http://www.yahoo.com/Health/Nutrition**

Newsgroups

Usenet:
   newsgroup: **sci.med.nutrition**
   newsgroup: **clari.biz.industry.food**
   newsgroup: **alt.support.diet**
   newsgroup: **alt.support.obesity**
   newsgroup: **alt.support.big-folks**
   newsgroup: **rec.food.veg**

Listservers

COMMNUTR-L (Community Nutrition)
   To join, send an e-mail to **lisproc@cornell.edu** with **sub commnutr-l
   <first name> <last name>** in the body of the message.

Food-for-thought (mailing list)
   To join, send an e-mail to **mailbase@mailbase.ac.uk** with **join food-for-
   thought <first name> <last name>** in the body of the message.

NUTEPI (Nutritional epidemiology)
>To join, send mail to **listserv@TUBVM.CS.TU-BERLIN.DE** with **sub NUTEPI <first name> <last name>** in the body of the message.

PHNUTR-L (Public health nutrition service providers)
>To join, send an e-mail to **listproc@u.washington.edu** with **sub phnutr-l <first name> <last name>** in the body of the message.

Occupational Health

Association for Worksite Health Promotion

Information related to programs, conferences, publications and the organization.

World Wide Web:
>URL: **http://www.awhp.com**

Canadian Centre for Occupational Health and Safety

Offers links to information and advice about occupational health and safety.

World Wide Web:
>URL: **http://www.ccohs.ca/**

Computers & Health

Offers information on ergonomics, carpal tunnel syndrome and VDT radiation.

Gopher:
>URL: **gopher://howler.ucs.indiana.edu:70/11/ Services/pubs/5_genintro/126health**

Computers and Health Web Page

Contains information about computer safety issues and pointers to safety guidelines for computer use. It also has a searchable index

World Wide Web:
>URL: **http://www-penninfo.upenn.edu:1962/ tiserve.mit.edu/9000/25204.html**

Injury Control Resource Information Network

Offers data, statistics, injury specific resources, research, publications and announcements of up-coming conferences

World Wide Web:
    URL: **http://www.pitt.edu/~1crin**

Occupational Safety and Health

Extensive on-line articles and documents concerning a variety of occupational
health risks and injuries. Also links to other resources.

World Wide Web:
    URL: **http://www.mic.ki.se/Safety.html**

OSHWEB

This is THE place to begin searching this topic. Information provided related to
chemical safety, emergency management, ergonomics, international organizations, hazard control, product safety, radiation, risk management, research institutes and publications. Searchable.

World Wide Web:
    URL: **http://turva.me.tut.fi/~OSHWEB/**

Newsgroups

Usenet:
    newsgroup: **comp.human.factors**
    newsgroup: **comp.risks**
    newsgroup: **sci.med.occupational**

Pharmacy

PharmInfoNet

Offers links to the publication "Medical Sciences Bulletin", articles, meeting
highlights, drug data, and patient information. There are also links to archives
from the **sci.med.pharmacy** newsgroup, a PharmMall with links to the home

pages of manufacturers, publishers and software developers, and a Pharmacy Corner devoted to the needs of practicing pharmacists.

World Wide Web:
    URL: **http://pharminfo.com**

PharmWeb Home Page

Provides links to a PharmWeb Directory for finding people, PharmWeb Appointments, posing vacancies in pharmacy and related professions, pharmacy related academic institutions and companies, government information, societies and groups and conferences and meetings. There is also a link to the newsgroups identified below.

World Wide Web:
    URL: **http://www.pharmweb.net**

University of Maryland Drug Information Service

A "submit a question" forum is a key element of this useful site. Also offers FAQ's on specific drug groups such as weight loss products, lithium, antidepressants and homeopathic remedies.

World Wide Web:
    URL: **http://www.pharmacy.ab.umd.edu/~umdi/umdi.html**

The "Virtual" Pharmacy Centre

Includes information about and links to drug databases, drug research and development, drug interactions, reactions and infusion rates, new drugs, drug alerts, clinical pharmacology and toxicology and links to associations and schools.

World Wide Web:
    URL: **http://www.sci.lib.uci.edu/~Martindale/Pharmacy.html/**

Newsgroups

Usenet:
    newsgroup: **sci.med.pharmacy**
    newsgroup: **sci.bio**
    newsgroup: **sci.bio.microbiology**

newsgroup. **sci.bio.technology**
newsgroup: **sci.chem**
newsgroup: **sci.med**
newsgroup: **sci.polymers**

Listservers

PHARM

To join, send mail to **PHARM-REQUEST@DMU.ac.uk** with **subscribe PHARM <first name> <last name>** in the body of the message.

Polio

Polio Survivors Page: Polio and Post-Polio Resources

Links to articles, information packets, newsletters and general resources related to Polio and Post-Polio Syndrome. A good place to start searching this topic.

World Wide Web:
URL: **http://www.eskimo.com/~dempt/polio.html**

Post-Polio Syndrome & Disabilities Resources

This site has on-line articles related to adaptations for daily living, rehabilitation and treatment, and causes and symptoms of Post-Polio Syndrome. Also links to support groups and home pages.

World Wide Web:
URL: **http://www.azstarnet.com/~rspear/**

Newsgroups

Usenet:
newsgroup: **alt.support.post-polio**

Rehabilitation

InContiNet

Provides general information for the public, full-text articles, abstracts and research designed for health care professionals, instrumentation information, and a listing of related professional and non-profit organizations.

World Wide Web:
URL: **http://www.IncontiNet.com/**

MedWeb: Physical Medicine and Rehabilitation

A comprehensive directory of links to a variety of rehab-related topics such as assistive technology, sports medicine, stroke, other Internet resources related to brain injury, cognitive rehabilitation, neurology, spinal chord injury, orthopedics, and patient education

World Wide Web:
URL: **http://www.gen.emory.edu/medweb.rehab.html**

Listservers

Incontilist (related to incontinence)
To join, send mail to **incontilist-list@Incontinet**.com with **subscribe Incontilist <first name> <last name>** in the body of the message.

REHAB-RU
To join, send mail to **listserv@ukcc.uky.edu** with **subscribe REHAB-RU <first name> <last name>** in the body of the message.

Repetitive Stress Injury

Computer-Related Repetitive Strain Injury (RSI)

Offers information on RSI, including links to other Web sites, including one with animations of stretches to do!

World Wide Web:
URL: **http://engr-www.unl.edu/ee/eeshop/rsi.html**

CTDNews

CTDNews current issue, prevention products, general information and bulletin board.

World Wide Web:
　　URL: **http://ctdnews.com**

ErgoWeb

Offers volumes of useful ergonomics information including instructional materials, standards and guidelines, news and products

World Wide Web:
　　URL: **http://www.ergoweb.com/Pub/ewhome.shtml**

Occupational Safety and Health Administration (OSHA)

Provides statistics and data, standards and technical information

World Wide Web:
　　URL: **http://www.osha.gov**

Typing Injuries FAQS and Links

Has links to general information about typing injuries, ergonomics, publications, references and keyboard alternatives. Another good beginning search site.

World Wide Web:
　　URL: **http://www.cs.princeton.edu/~dwallach/tifaq**

Typing Injuries Web Page

Has links to many other sources of repetitive strain injury(RSI) information, on-line information about a variety of RSIs including carpal tunnel syndrome, tendonitis, and thoracic outlet syndrome, FAQ's and the RSI Newsletter. There are also links to information about treatments, adaptive technologies and product literature and reviews.

World Wide Web:
　　URL: **http://alumni.caltech.edu/~dank/typing-archive.html**

Research

International Health Care Research Guide

Provides an international health care researcher database to enable you to communicate with other researchers with similar interests. Also offers links to other health research sites.

World Wide Web:
   URL: **http://www.health.ucalgary.ca/**

National Institute of Nursing Research (NINR)

This site offers several documents including the National Nursing Research Agenda. Of greatest interest is the list of current program announcements and requests for applications. Guidelines for various grants and traineeships are also included.

World Wide Web:
   URL: **http://www.nih.gov/ninr/**

National Institutes of Health: Scientific Resources

Provides research news, research training information and listings of NIH research projects and sites

World Wide Web:
   URL: **http://www.nih.gov/science**

Research Institutes

A vast collection of links to reseach institues related to a variety of health topics.

World Wide Web:
   URL: **http://pie.org/E21224T3783**

Newsgroups

Usenet:
    newsgroup: **sci.research**

Sexual Assault

Rape and Sexual Assault Resources

A good starting place to browse for links related to this topic.

World Wide Web:
    URL: **http://www.crl.com/~thefly/abuse/rapeandsexassault.html**

Sexual Assault Information Page

Provides links to articles related to families, child sexual abuse, rape, sexual harassment, incest, domestic violence, prevention and law.

World Wide Web:
    URL: **http://www.cs.utk.edu/~bartley/saInfoPage.html**

Sexuality

Sex Info

Contains articles on healthy sex, birth control, disease/pregnancy prevention, and sexually transmitted diseases.

World Wide Web:
    URL: **http://www.uiuc.edu/departments/mckinley/health-info/ sexual/sexual.html**

Yahoo Safe Sex WWW Page

Offers links to information on birth control, condoms, male contraceptives and safe-sex manuals.

World Wide Web:
    URL: **http://www.yahoo.com/Society_and_Culture/Sexuality/
    Activities_and_Practices/Safe_Sex/**

Newsgroups

Usenet:
    newsgroup: **alt.sex**

Sleep

SleepNet's Guide

Offers information about a variety of sleep disorders, sleep deprivation, sleep-
related products, a listing of sleep disorder centers and support groups and extensive links to other sites.

World Wide Web:
    URL: **http://www.sleepnet.com**

Sleep Medicine Home Page

Provides links to newsgroups, FAQ's, articles and text files, and other Internet
sites related to sleep. Many of these resources relate to children's sleep problems and SIDS

World Wide Web:
    URL: **http://www.cloud9.net:80/~thorpy/**

Phantom Sleep Page

Incorporates the patient directed site S.N.O.R.E., that provides links to information on sleep disorders including obstructive sleep disorder and the procedure
Laser-Assisted Uvulopalatoplasty. Also a sleep disorders FAQ, information on
sleep apnea and snoring for both the public and health care professionals.

World Wide Web:
    URL: **http://www.newtechpub.com/phantom/**

Newsgroups

Usenet:
    newsgroup: **alt.support.sleep-disorder**

Smoking

CDC's Tobacco Information & Prevention (TIPS) Sourcepage

Includes full-text articles, data, reports and statistics related to tobacco use by a variety of specific populations. Also includes a publication list, a public information section on "how to quit" , other educational materials and a search facility.

World Wide Web:
    URL: **http://www.cdc.gov/nccdphp/osh/tobacco.htm**

CRISP (Computer Retrieval of Information on Scientific Projects)

Provides a gopher menu with over 200 items related to smoking cessation

Gopher:
    URL: **gopher://gopher.nih.gov/77/gopherlib/**
    indices/localmenu/index?smoking +cessation

National Clearinghouse on Tobacco and Health

Provides full-text articles on a variety of tobacco-related issues for the public and health professional, including a youth series, and environmental tobacco smoke series. Also includes searchable databases of conferences, Web documents and selected useful Websites.

World Wide Web:
    URL: **http://fox.nstn.ca/~ncth2/index.html**

NicNet: Arizona Nicotine and Tobacco Network

Offers extensive links to information and searches related to smoking and smoking cessation, tobacco advertising, and other web sites.

World Wide Web:
    URL: **http://ahsc.arizona.edu/nicnet**

Nursing Center for Tobacco Intervention

Features research abstracts, resource lists and intervention guidelines

World Wide Web:
    URL: **http://www.con.ohio-state.edu/tobacco**

U.S. Food & Drug Administration :Children and Tobacco

Includes fact sheets and full-text documents related to FDA's regulation of to-bacco products

World Wide Web:
    URL: **http://www.fda.gov/opacom/campaigns/tobacco.html**

Newsgroups

Usenet:
    newsgroup: **clari.news.smoking**
    newsgroup: **alt.support.stop-smoking**
    newsgroup: **alt.support.non-smokers**
    newsgroup: **alt.support.non-smokers (moderated)**
    newsgroup: **alt.smokers**

Listserv

    List: address: **smoke-free@msstate.edu**
    Subscription address: **smoke-free-request@msstate.edu**
    List address: **on-listproc@msstate.edu**
    Subscription address: **on-listproc-request@msstate.edu**

Spirituality

IHP-NET: International Network for Interfaith Health Practices

Provides links to information about the relationship between spirituality and health, the congregational nurse program and other related sites.

World Wide Web:
URL: **http://interaccess.com**

Listservers

Interfaith Health Practices
To join, send mail to **MAJORDOMO@interaccess.com** with **subscribe IHP-NET** in the body of the message.

Stress

Stress

Provides sub menus related to stress management techniques aimed at the general public.

World Wide Web:
URL: **http://www.uiuc.edu/departments/mckinley/health-info/stress /stress. html**

Stroke

National Stroke Association

Provides on-line information for the public and professionals related to stroke prevention, screening, treatment and research.

World Wide Web:
URL: **http://www.stroke.org/index.html**

Stroke: Internet Resources

This site has good links to a variety of articles, associations, practice guidelines and research related to stroke.

World Wide Web:
    URL: **http://views.vcu.edu/html/pmr/trowland/pted/cvawww.html**

WWW Stroke Resources: A Guide for Health Care Professionals

Offers links to clinical sites, education, anatomy, patient guides, organizations, stroke prevention and neurological evaluation instruments.

World Wide Web:
    URL: **http://griffin.vcu.edu/html/pmr/other/stroke.html**

Listservers

STROKE-L
    To join, send mail to **listserv@ukcc.uky.edu** with **subscribe STROKE-L <first name> <last name>** in the body of the message.

Sudden Infant Death Syndrome

The Canadian Foundation for the Study of Infant Deaths

Provides information about SIDS, available resources and other sites, including a French version.

World Wide Web:
    URL: **http://www.sidscanada.org/sids.html**

National Sudden Infant Death Syndrome Resource Center

Provides information sheets and publications, annotated bibliographies, an information exchange newsletter and reference and referral services.

World Wide Web:
    URL: **http://www.ichp.ufl.edu/MCH-NetLink/SIDS/SIDS1.htm**

SIDS Network

Includes full-text articles about SIDS in English, Spanish and German, information about support groups, research information and links to other resources.

World Wide Web:
    URL: **http://sids-network.org**

Sudden Infant Death Syndrome

Offers general information about SIDS. It is sometimes difficult to contact.

Gopher:
    URL: **gopher://gopher.vifp.monash.edu.au:70/11/Medical/sids**

Wellness

Cyberspace Wellness Center

Provides on-line health screening questionnaires, links to prevention services, and links to other resources. Interesting presentation, but not a lot of substance.

World Wide Web:
    URL: **http://www.telemedical.com/~drcarr/Telemedical/cws.html**

Wellness, Health & Fitness on the Internet

Provides a good set of links to a variety of wellness resources and articles.

World Wide Web:
    URL: **http://pages.ripco.com:8080/~awhp/links.html**

Wellness Links

Offers links to a wide variety of wellness resources including holistic and alternative practices,

World Wide Web:
    URL: **http://www.wellmedia.com/links.html**

WellnessWeb

Provides information related to a variety of wellness topics, including stress management, women's health, smoker's clinic, cancer center and senior's center. Also links to a variety of disease/condition-specific mailing lists.

World Wide Web:
    URL: **http://wellweb.com**

Listservers

Wellnesslist
    To join, send mail to **majordomo@wellnessmart.com** with **subscribe Wellnesslist <first name> <last name>** in the body of the message.

Women's Health

National Institutes of Health

Offers links to information relating to health issues and clinical protocols, research, special interest groups, the NIH Library and other Internet resources.

World Wide Web:
    URL: **http://www.nih.gov/**

The Virtual Hospital

Provides links to a variety of teaching materials including multimedia textbooks, multimedia teaching files, patient simulations/virtual patients, lectures and patient-related material.

World Wide Web:
    URL: **http://vh.radiology.uiowa.edu:80/**

University of Michigan Clearinghouse of Resource Guides

Provides links to resource guides on a large variety of health-related and other topics. A good browsing site!

World Wide Web:
    URL: **http://http2.sils.umich.edu/~lou/chhome.html**
    URL: **http://www.lib.umich.edu/chhome.html**

Gopher:
   URL: **gopher://una.hh.lib.umich.edu/11/inetdirs**

Women's Health

Provides extensive information on women's health topics including breast self-exam, cryotherapy, menstrual cramps, pap test, colposcopy, pelvic inflammatory disease, pre-menstrual syndrome, pregnancy, toxic shock syndrome, and urinary tract infection.

World Wide Web:
   URL: **http://www.uiuc.edu/departments/mckinley/health-info/ womenhlt/women**

Women's Health

Provides links to information about women's emotional, physical and sexual health. Information about eating disorders, pregnancy, and menopause are included.

World Wide Web:
   URL: **http://www.lib.umich.edu/chdocs/ womenhealth/womens_health.html**

World Health Organization

Includes information about major programs, World Health Report, Weekly Epidemiological Record, WHO's Statistical Information System, World Health Day, public information, newsletters, and international travel requirements and advice.

World Wide Web:
   URL: **http://www.who.org**

Gopher:
   URL: **gopher://gopher.who.org**

Telnet
   Address: **lynx.who.ch**
   Login: **www**

Listservers

HMATRIX-L (concerning on-line health resources)
> To join, send mail to **listserv@ukanaix.cc.ukans.edu** with **subscibe HMATRIX-L <first name> <last name>** in the body of the message.

Online Journals

Alternative Medicine Digest

World Wide Web:
> URL: **http://www.alternativemedicine.com/digest.html**

The American Nurse

World Wide Web:
> URL: **http://www.nursingworld.org/pubs.htm**

AMIA Nursing Informatics Working Group Newsletters

World Wide Web:
> URL: **http://www.gl.umbc.edu/~abbott/letters.htm**

Arthritis Today

World Wide Web:
> URL: **http://www.enews.com/at**

Australian Electronic Journal of Nursing Education (AEJNE)

World Wide Web:
> URL: **http://www.csu.edu.au/aejnehp.htm**

Bandolier: Evidence-based health care

World Wide Web:
> URL: **http://www.jr2.ox.ac.uk/Bandolier/**

Chronic Immune Dysfunction Syndrome Quarterly

Gopher:
URL: **gopher.enews.com/cidsq**

Computers in Nursing Interactive

World Wide Web:
URL: **http://www.cini.com/cin**

Diabetes Self Management

World Wide Web:
URL: **http://www.enews/diabetes**

Disability International

World Wide Web:
URL: **http://www.escape.ca/di.html**

Harvard Public Health Review

World Wide Web:
URL: **http://biosun1.harvard.edu/hphr.html**

Health After Fifty (Johns Hopkins medical newsletter)

World Wide Web:
URL: **http://www.enews.com/jhml**

Health and Medical Informatics Digest

World Wide Web:
URL: **http://maddog.fammed.wisc.edu/hmid.html**

HIV: An Electronic Media Information Review

World Wide Web:
URL: **http://florey.biosci.uq.edu.au/hiv/NURSING/nursing.htm**

IMIA Newsletters

World Wide Web:
    URL: **http://www.cqu.edu.au/healthsci/**
          profassoc/imia/imiahome.htm#imia

Internurse: A Resource for Nurses and Midwives

World Wide Web:
    URL: **http://www.wp.com:80/InterNurse**

Journal of the American Medical Association

World Wide Web:
    URL: **http://www.ama-assn.org/amahome.htm**

Journal of Epidemiology and Community Health

World Wide Web:
    URL: **http://info.mcc.ac.uk/JECH**

The Lancet

World Wide Web:
    URL: **http://www.thelancet.com**

The Maternal/Child Nursing Journal

World Wide Web:
    URL: **http://www.ajn.org/page1.html**

Medical Sciences Bulletin

World Wide Web:
    URL: **http://www.pharminfo.com/pubs/msb/msbmnu.html**

Mental Health Net-Perspectives

World Wide Web:
URL: **http://www.cmhm.com/perspectives/**

New England Journal of Medicine

World Wide Web:
URL: **http://www.nejm.org**

Nursing Connections

World Wide Web:
URL: **http://nursing-www.mc.duke.edu:80/nursing/nsgconx.htm**

Nurseweek

World Wide Web:
URL: **http://www.nurseweek.com**

Nursing Research

World Wide Web:
URL: **http://www.ajn.org/page1.html**

Nursing Standard Online

World Wide Web:
URL: **http://www.nursing-standard.co.uk/nso.htm**

Nursing Trends and Issues

World Wide Web:
URL: **http://www.nursingworld.org/products/ntipromo.htm**

Nutrition Action Healthletter

World Wide Web:
URL: **http://www.enews.com/nah**

On-line Journal of Issues in Nursing

World Wide Web:
    URL: **http://www.nursingworld.org/ojin/ojinhome.htm**

On-line Journal of Nursing Informatics

World Wide Web:
    URL: **http://milkman.cac.psu.edu/~dxm12/OJNI.html**

Progress: A Readable Digest of New Cancer Treatments

Written for the public, editorial control by OncoLink.

World Wide Web:
    URL: **http://www.cancerprog.com**

Revista Rol De Enfermeria

World Wide Web:
    URL: **http://www.readysoft.es/rol**

Searchable Health-Related Literature Databases

Cinahl Direct

Cumulative Index to Nursing and Allied Health Literature. References over 900 journals. Output includes bibliographic data and abstracts. Paid membership required.

World Wide Web:
    URL: **http://www.cinahl.com/**

Medline

Requires a valid account. A list of vendors is found at this site.

World Wide Web:
    URL: **http://sils.umich.edu/~nscherer/Medline/MedlineGuide.html**

<u>Springhouse Reference Library</u>

References over 100 nursing journals. Output includes bibliographic data and abstracts. No membership required.

World Wide Web:
   URL: **http://www.springnet.com/journals.htm**

Glossary

Alias:

A special recipient name for a group of Internet addresses.

Anonymous FTP:

Computer site set to allow public retrieval of files using the login anonymous.

Archie:

An information retrieval system for anonymous FTP sites.

Backbone:

The basic communications link of a network.

Digest:

A collection of messages about a specific topic prepared by a mailing list moderator.

Domain name:

Name of a computer system that is registered with the Internet. Can be made up of sub-domains such as geographical or organizational sub-domains.

Dynamic rerouting:

Ability of a network to direct communications around a damaged connection to still reach the intended recipient.

E-mail:

Electronic mail

Emoticons:

Icons for indicating emotions.

FAQ

Frequently Asked Questions

Forum:

Same as a Newsgroup.

FreeNet:

A computer network that brings together the resources of a community or campus and is available free of charge.

FTP:

File Transfer Protocol, is a set of specifications that support Internet file transfer.

Gateway: Computer system that acts as a point of access that allows information to move back and forth between networks.

Gopher: A way of organizing and categorizing certain types of information on the Internet.

Host: A synonym for any computer, generally at a remote location.

Hypertext: Text that contains imbedded links to other data.

Internet: The name for a group of worldwide computer-based information resources connected together.

Jughead: An information retrieval system for a specific Gopher site.

Listserv: Listserver, the most common computerized mailing list administration program.

Login id: Unique identifying character string assigned to a user of a computer system.

Luddite: A person who believes that the progress brought by machines is dangerous to the public good.

Lurking: Listening in on a mailing list or newsgroup discussion without replying.

Lynx: A text-based Web Browser program.

Mailing list: A collection of Internet addresses that facilitates an electronic discussion group.

Mosaic: A windows-based Web Browser program

Netscape: A windows-based Web Browser program.

Network: Two or more computers connected together so that information can move between them.

Newsgroup: A collecting site for messages about a specific theme

Newsreaders: Programs used to access a newsgroup, such as rn, tn, nn, and tin.

Password: String of characters secretly chosen to verify that you are the valid user connected with a specific userid

PPP: Point to Point Protocol

SLIP: Serial Line Internet Protocol

TCP / IP: Transmission Control Protocol/Internet protocol

Telnet: A program used to connect to a remote computer.

**Terminal emulation   The process that allows your computer screen and
connection:**   keyboard to control a remote computer.

URL: Uniform Resource Locator, a standardized method
                                  for referencing an item on the World Wide Web, in-
                                  cluding a complete description and its location.

Usenet: User's Network, made up of all machines that receive
                                  network newsgroups.

Userid: User identification, synonymous with login id.

Veronica: An information retrieval system for Gopher sites.

WAIS: Wide Area Information Servers, a way of categoriz-
                                  ing and organizing certain types of information on
                                  the Internet.

Web Browser: An information retrieval program for the World
                                  Wide Web that can interpret and display hypertext
                                  documents.

Index